Courage
Over
Cancer

David J. Reimer Sr.

Crave Press

Dedication

This book is dedicated to those who have fought the battle with cancer, to their caregivers, and to their support systems.

You are the embodiment of courage.

Introduction

Merriam Webster defines courage as "mental or moral strength to venture, persevere, and withstand danger, fear, or difficulty." Lions have been used to symbolize the ultimate courage needed to survive in the wilds of life, to overcome any obstacle and to survive triumphantly; however we all have the lion's spirit inside of us to overcome hardship. This spirit is evident in everyone fighting a battle with cancer.

Cancer survivors as well as those who have lost their battle have endured the physical and emotional effects of tests and treatments. Their positive attitude and their strength to persevere through their fear and physical ailments are true examples of courage.

This book presents a lightsome photographic journey of courage in the face of cancer with lions representing the emotional and physical highs and lows of the battle with cancer and the road to recovery.

"He is a man of courage who does not run away, but remains at his post and fights against the enemy."

~Socrates

. . . . .so it begins

Waiting to see the doctor

"Courage is doing what you're afraid to do. There can be no courage unless you're scared."

~Edward Vernon Rickenbacker

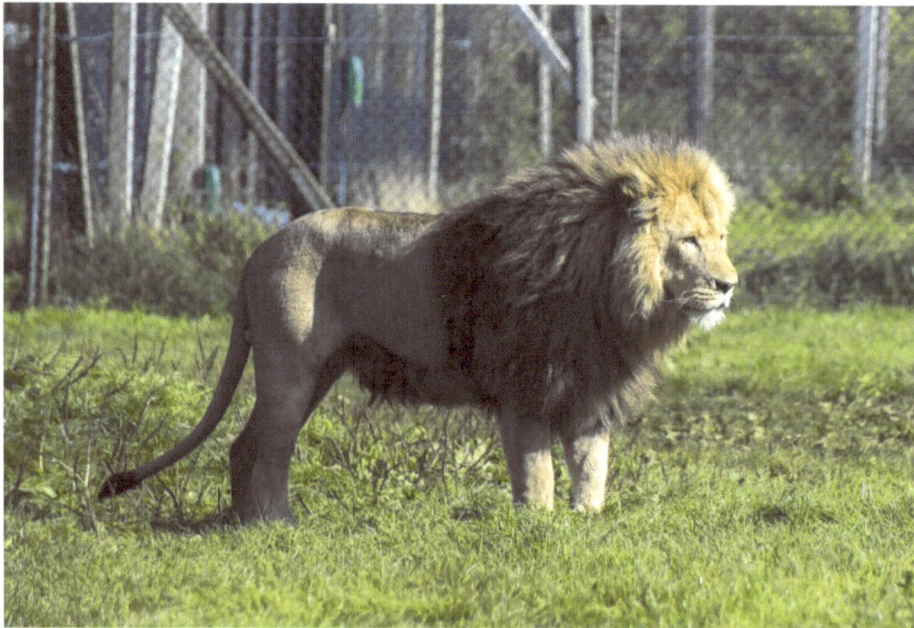

Waiting for test results

"Courage is fear holding on a minute longer."

~General George S. Patton Jr.

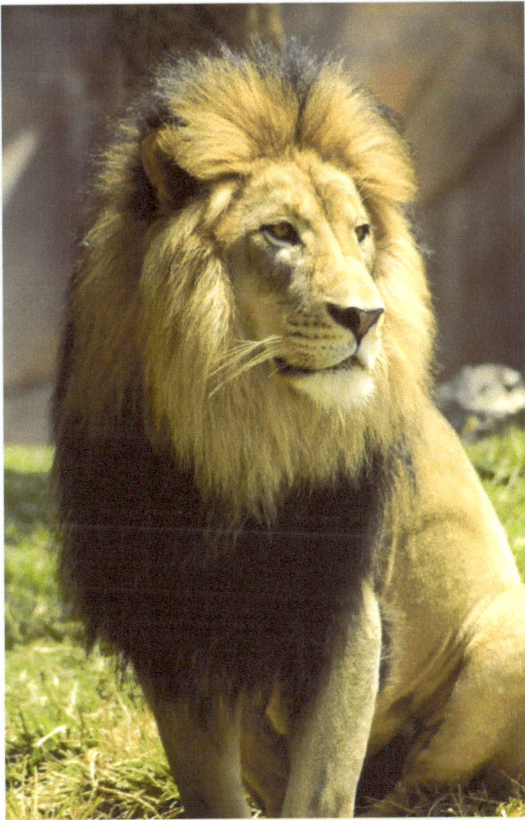

Treatment.......

..and what goes with it

Chemo

"There were times when chemo would eat my body, but I told myself that I have the strength and courage to win and come out stronger."

~Yuvraj Singh

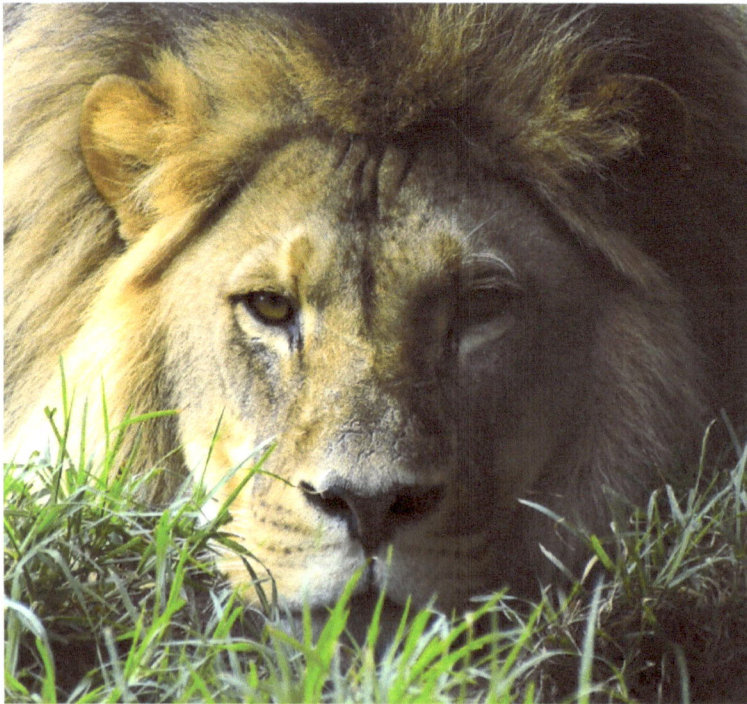

Radiation

(expect some tattoos)

"Courage, above all things, is the first quality of a warrior."

~Carl von Clausewitz

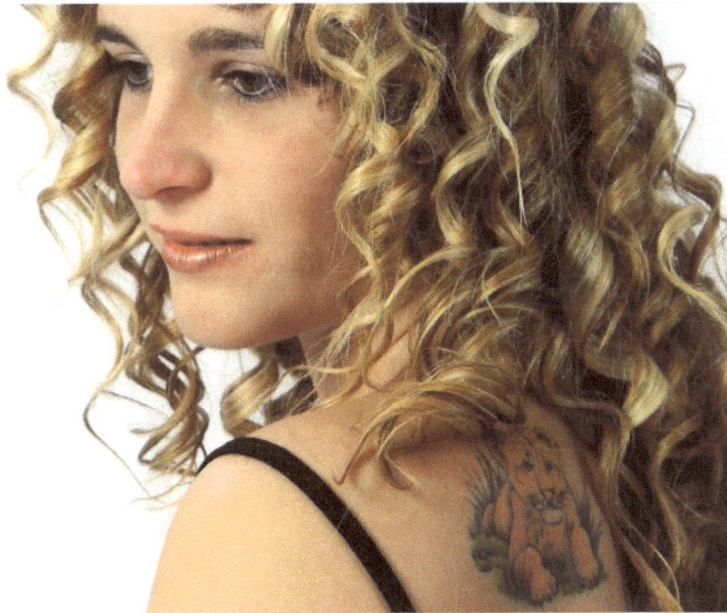

Loss of appetite, smell, and taste

"Courage is like love; it must have hope for nourishment."

~Napoleon Bonaparte

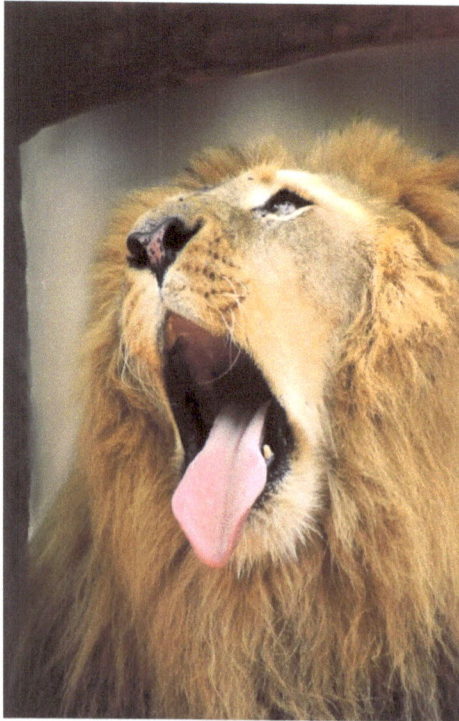

Hair loss

(whole body)

"Courage is as often the outcome of despair as of hope; in the one case we have nothing to lose, in the other everything to gain."

~Diane de Poitiers

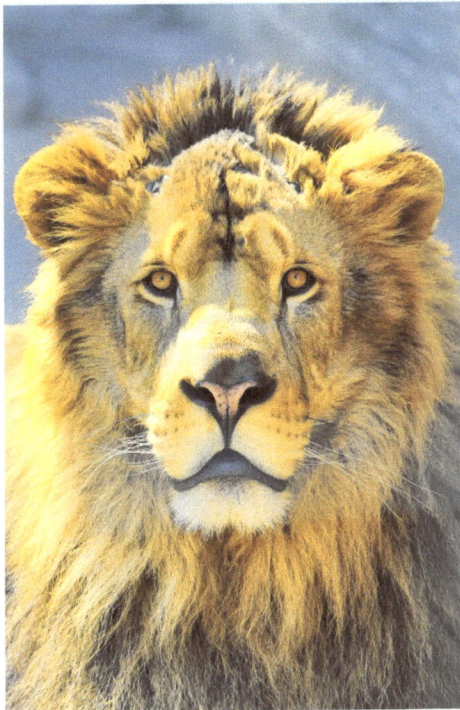

Hearing loss

"Be happy with what you have while working for what you want."

~Helen Keller

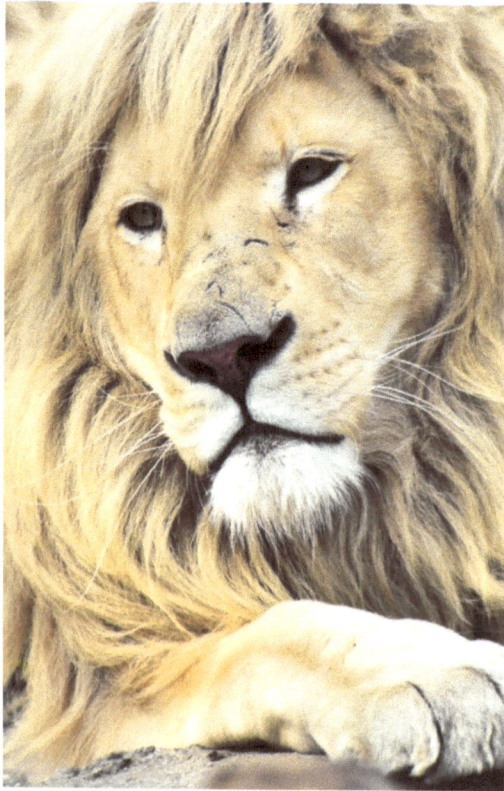

Weight loss

"Hope is being able to see that there is light despite all of the darkness."

~Desmond Tutu

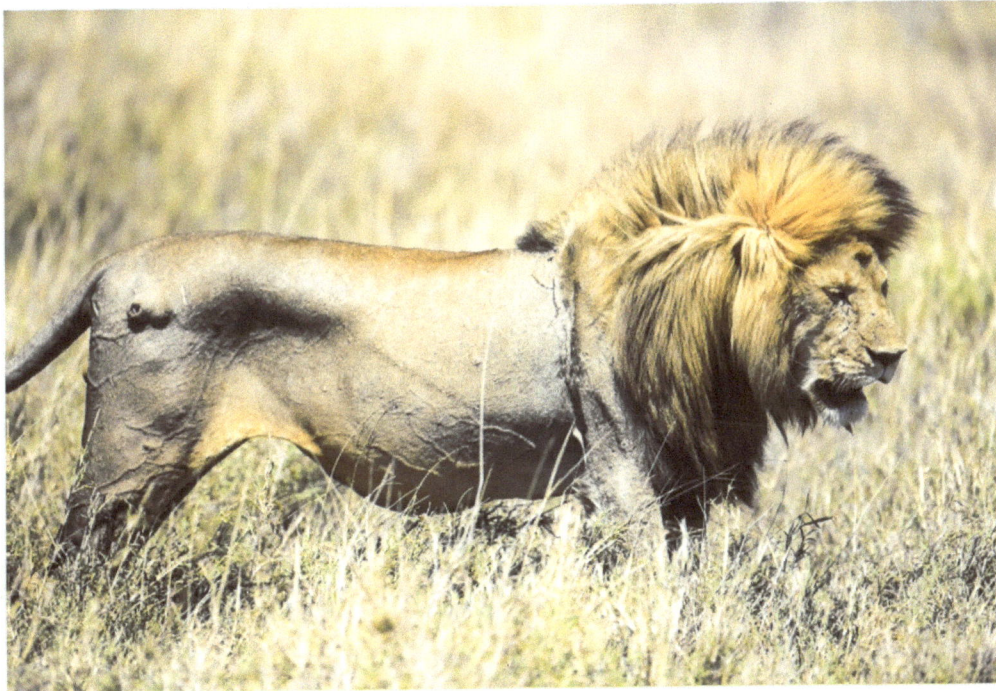

Dry mouth

"Man cannot discover new oceans unless he has the courage to lose sight of the shore."

~André Gide

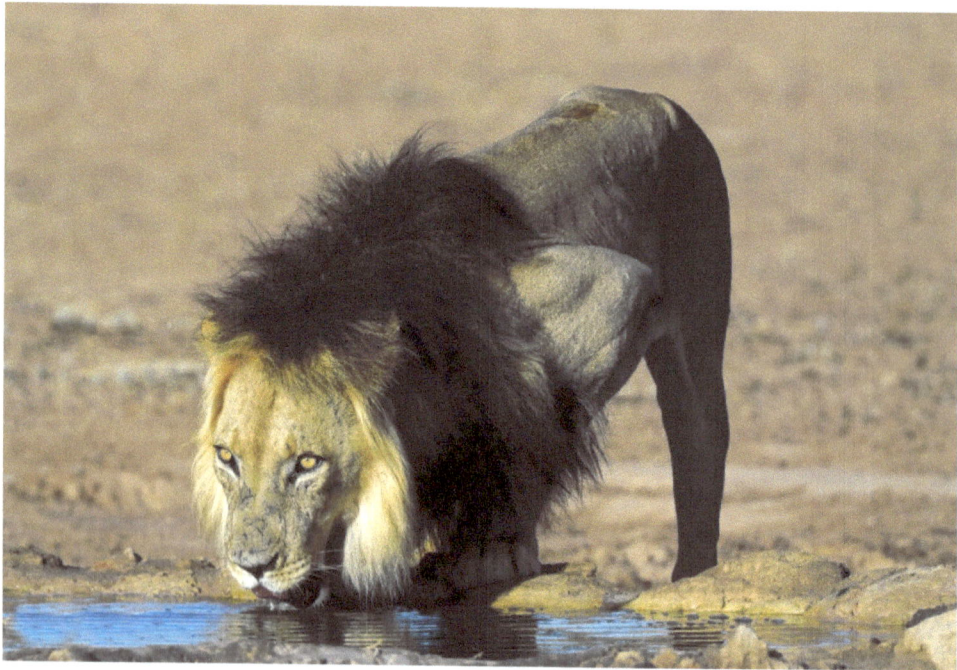

Mouth sores

"Pain is never permanent."

~Saint Teresa of Avila

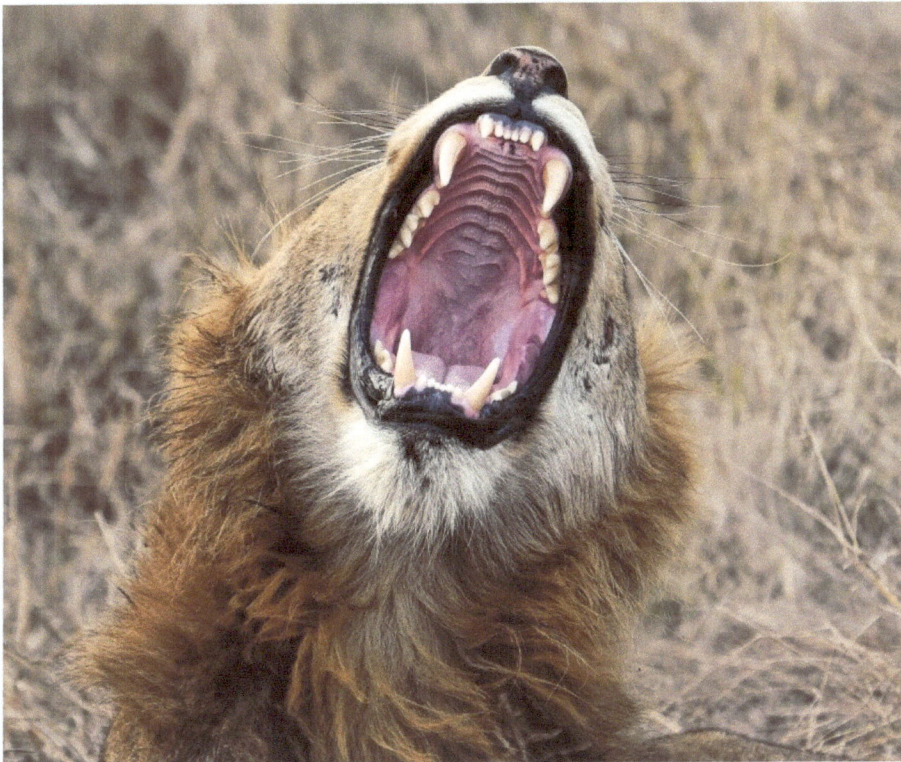

Decreased muscle mass
(loss of muscle tone)

"Courage is being scared to death but saddling up anyway."

~John Wayne

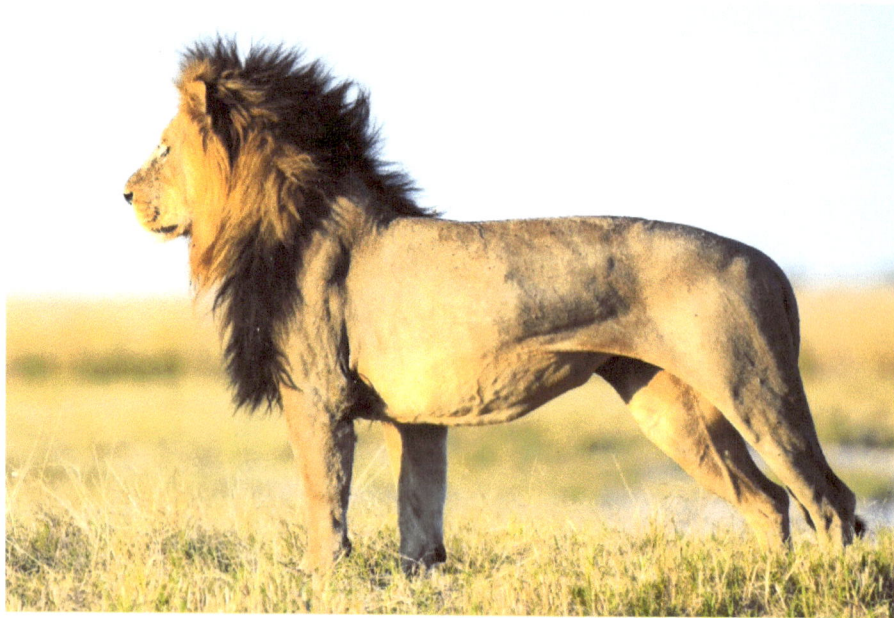

Fevers

"If you could get up the courage to begin, you have the courage to succeed."

~David Viscott

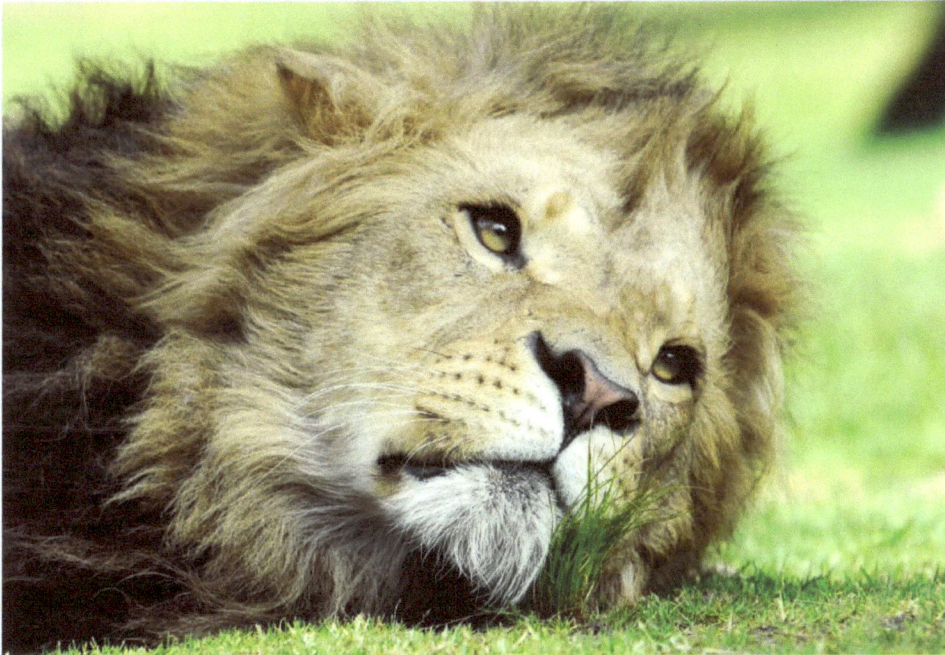

Fear of infections

"Courage is contagious. When a brave man takes a stand, the spines of others are often stiffened."

~Billy Graham

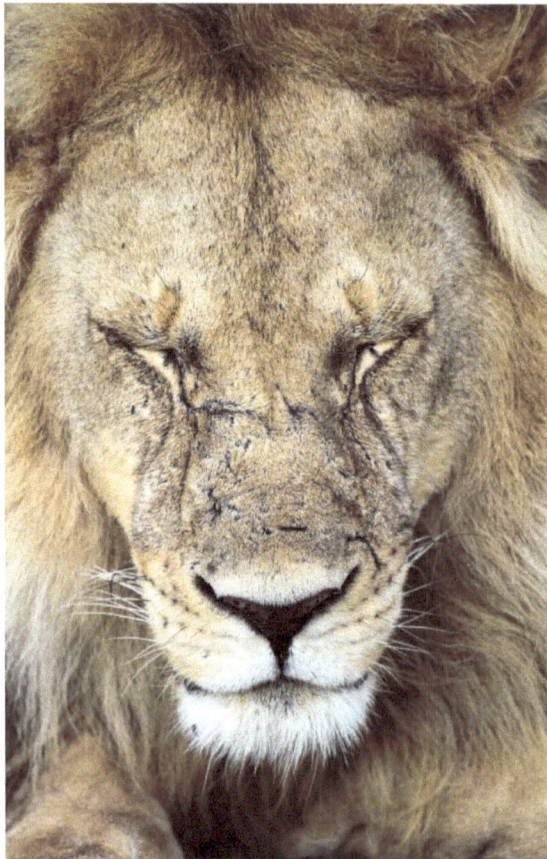

Nausea

"Healing takes courage, and we will have courage, even if we have to dig a little to find it."

~Tori Amos

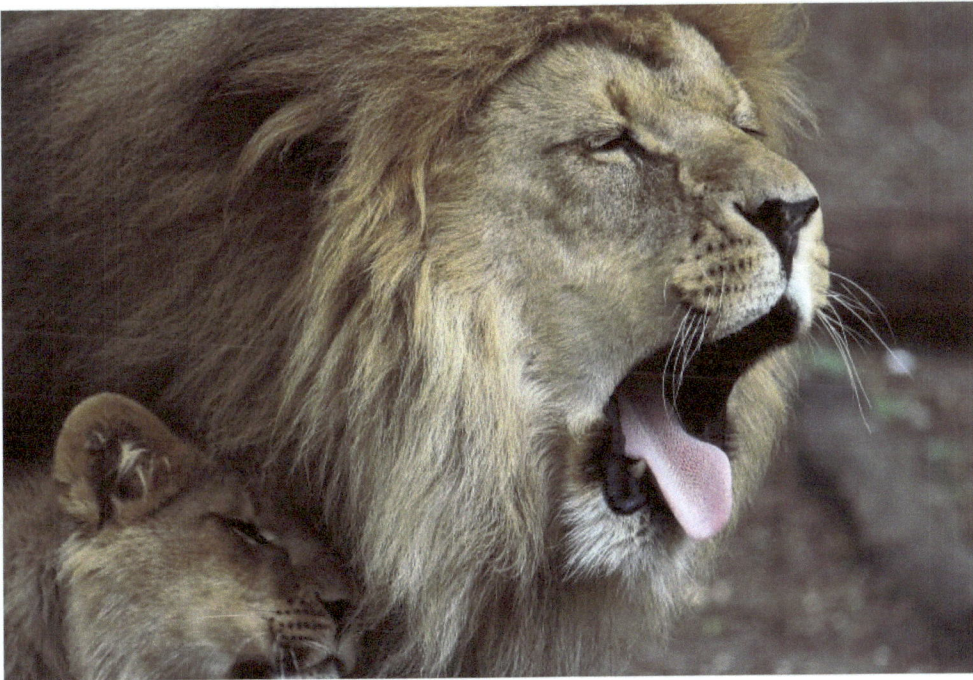

Concentration problems

"Courage – a perfect sensibility of the measure of danger, and a mental willingness to endure it."

~William Tecumseh Sherman

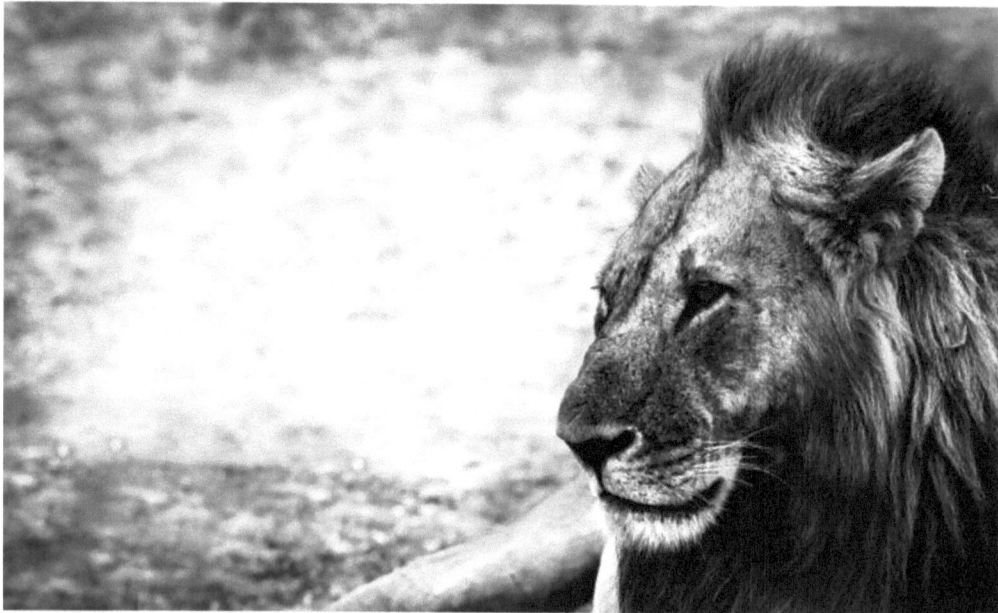

Heartburn and Indigestion

"Fear and courage are brothers."

~Proverb

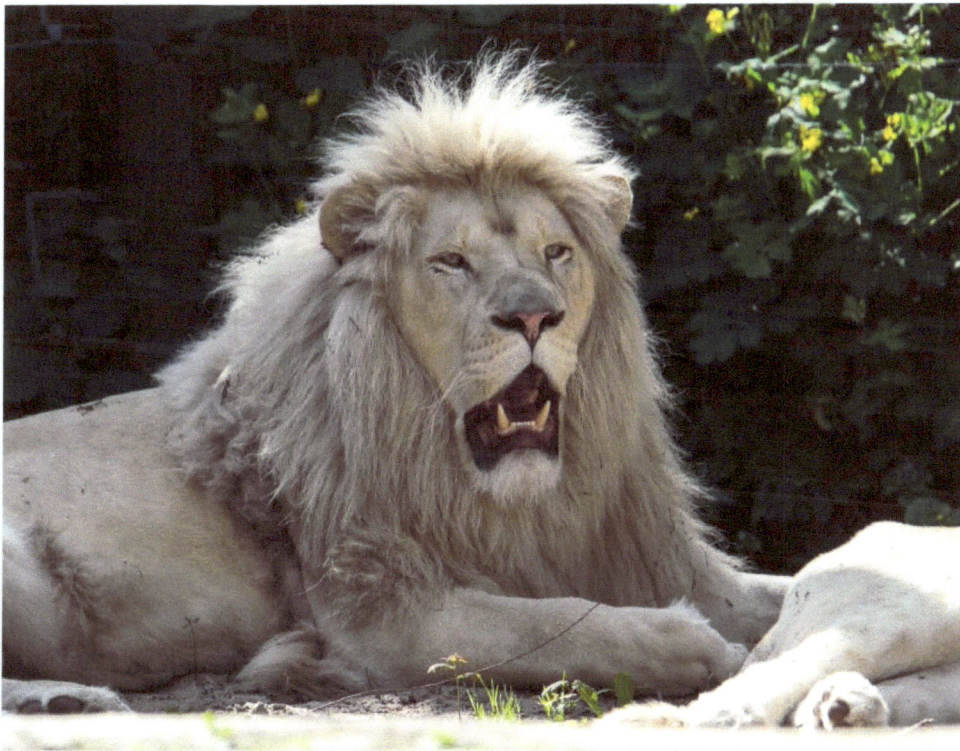

Bone pain

"If pain must come, may it come quickly. Because I have a life to live, and I need to live it in the best way possible."

~Paulo Coelho

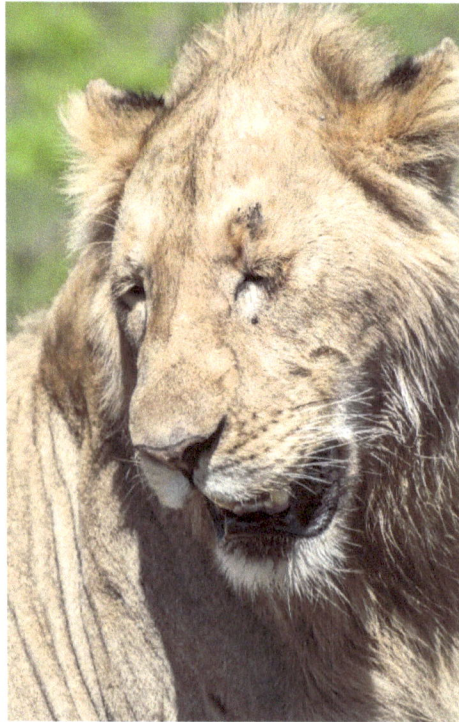

Dizziness

"Believe you can and you're halfway there."

~Theodore Roosevelt

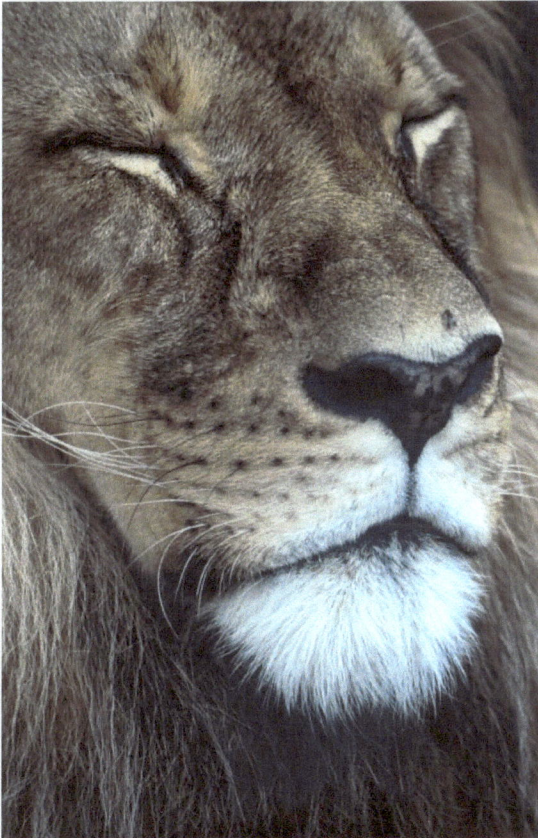

Feeling like a pin cushion

"Always be courageous and strong, and don't fear."

~Gabby Douglas

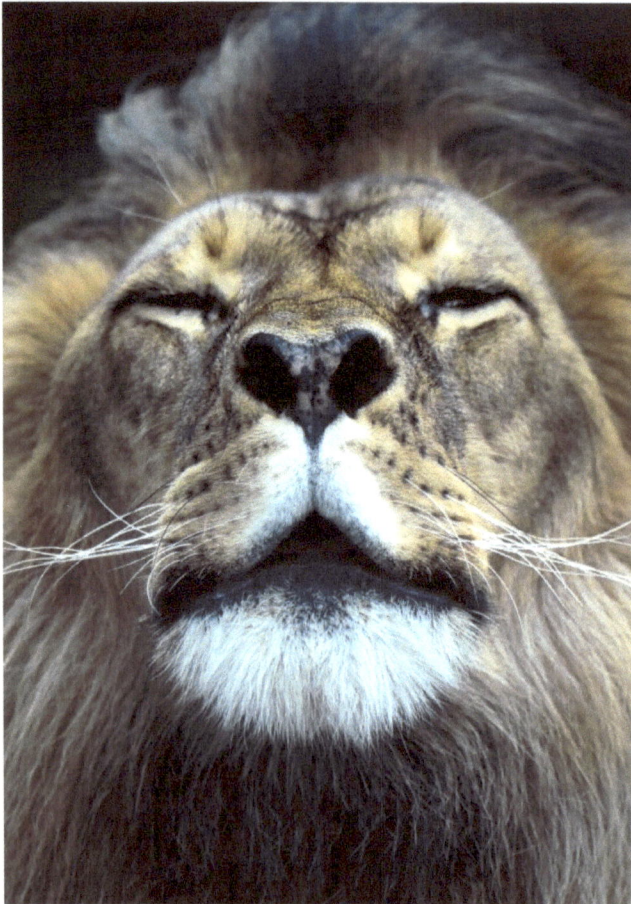

Nail pigment changes

"If your life changes, we can change the world, too."

~Yoko Ono

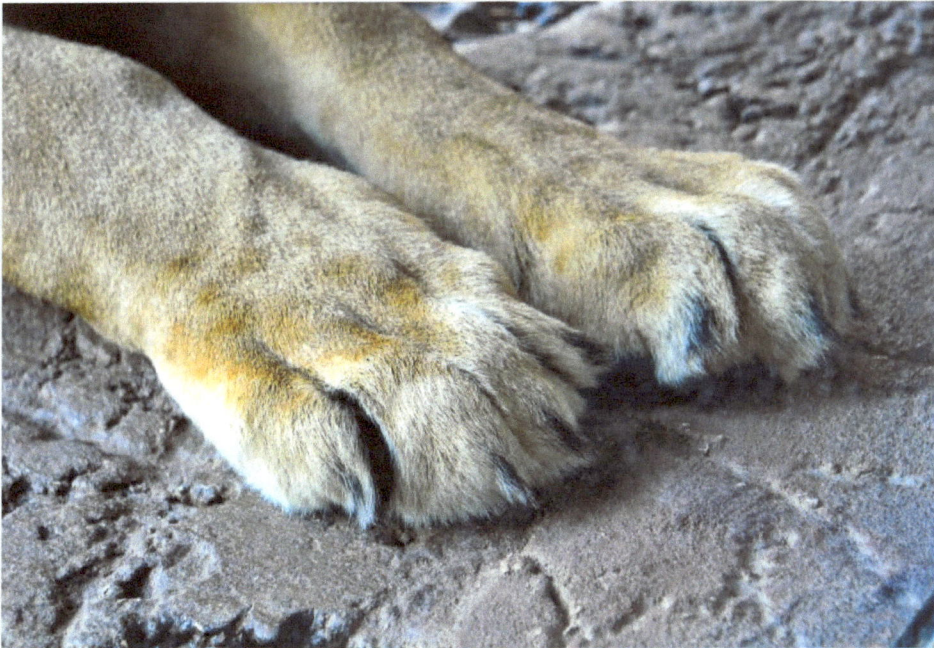

Anemia

"Courage is tiny pieces of fear all glued together."

~Terri Guillemets

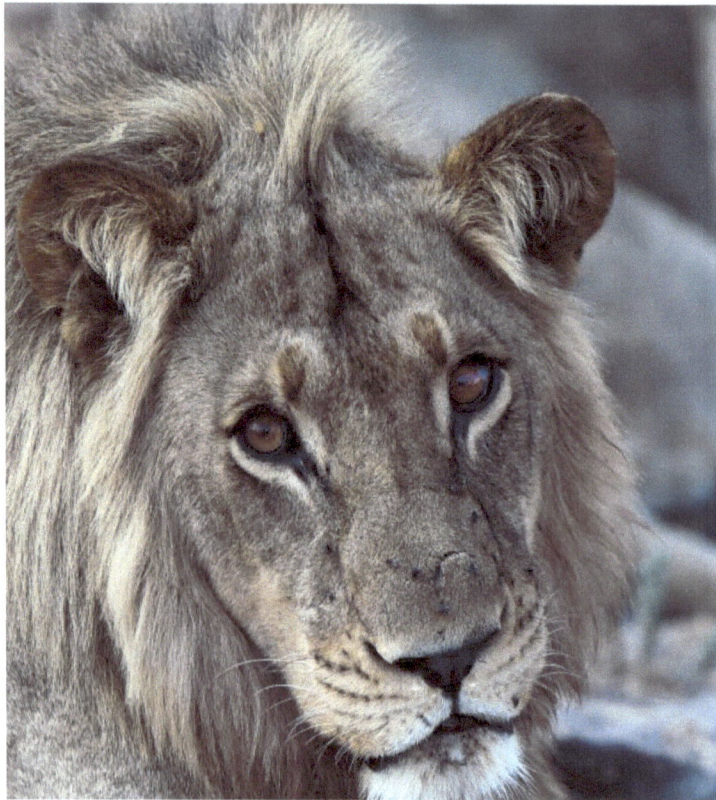

Bleeding and Bruising

"Every day you either see a scar or courage.
Where you dwell will define your struggle."

~Dodinsky

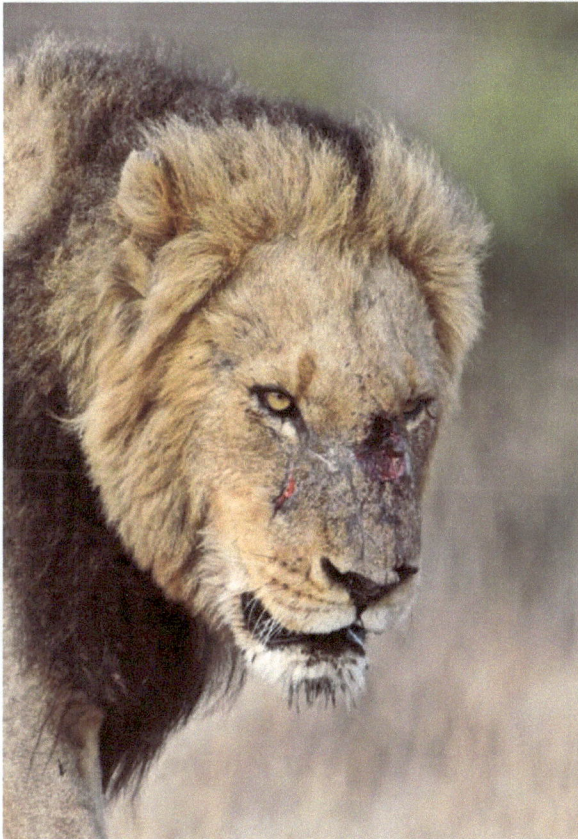

Insomnia

"I find hope in the darkest of days, and focus in the brightest. I do not judge the universe."

~Dalai Lama

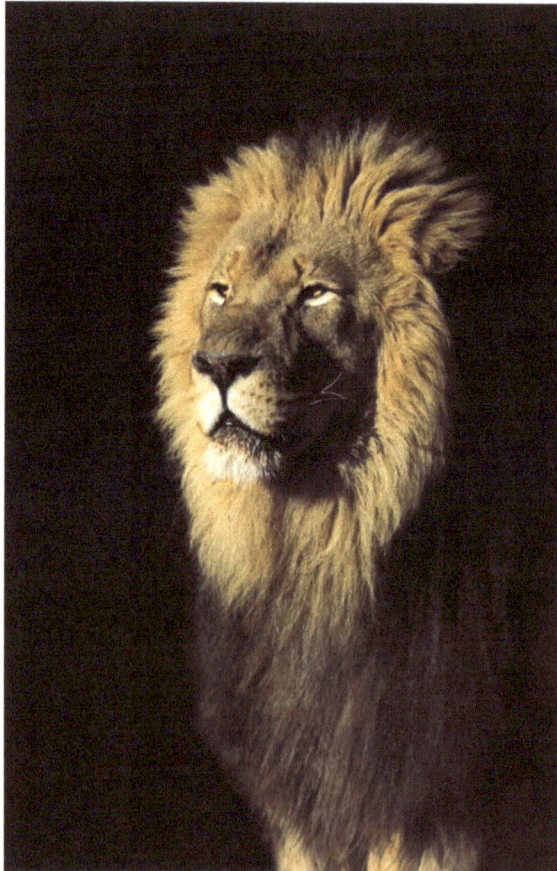

Night sweats
(chills & hot flashes)

"Courage is a peculiar kind of fear."

~Charles Kennedy

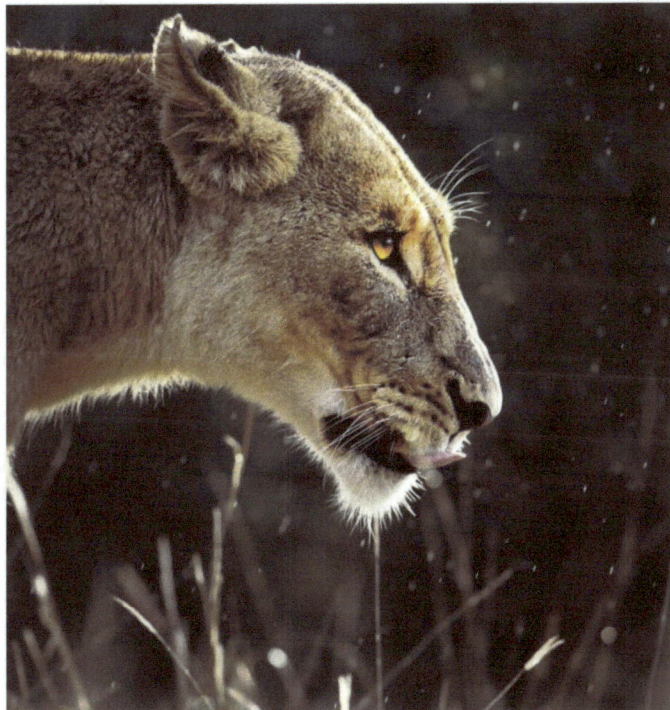

Chest pain or Heart races

"Who could refrain that had a heart to love and in that heart courage to make's love known?"

~William Shakespeare

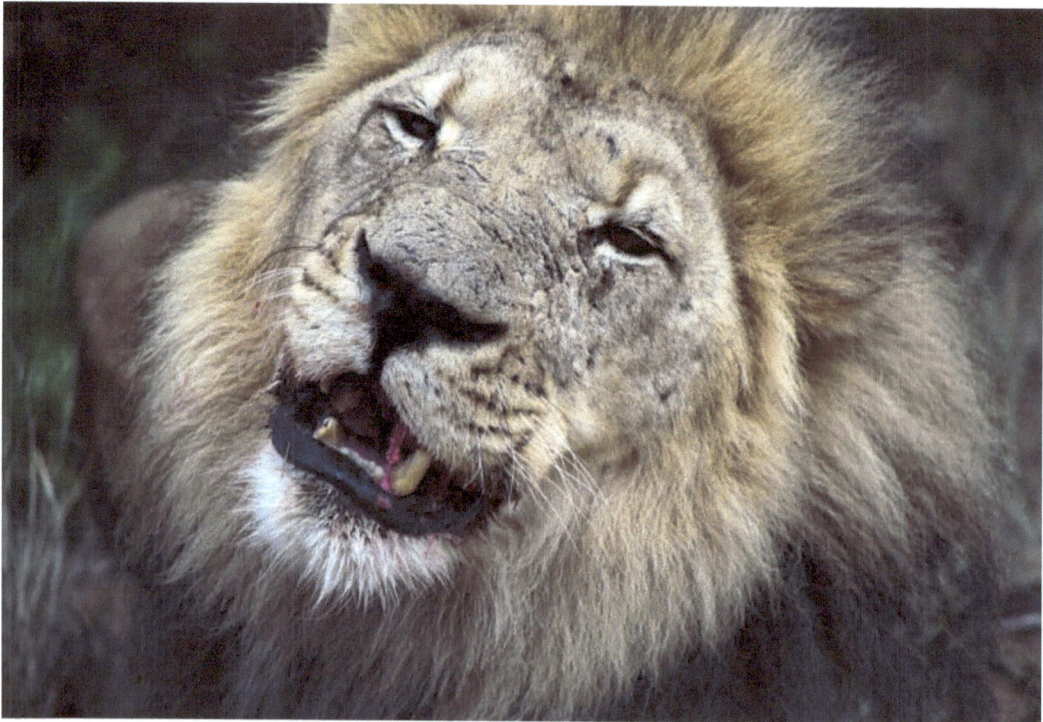

Diarrhea

"Health is not valued till sickness comes."

~Thomas Fuller

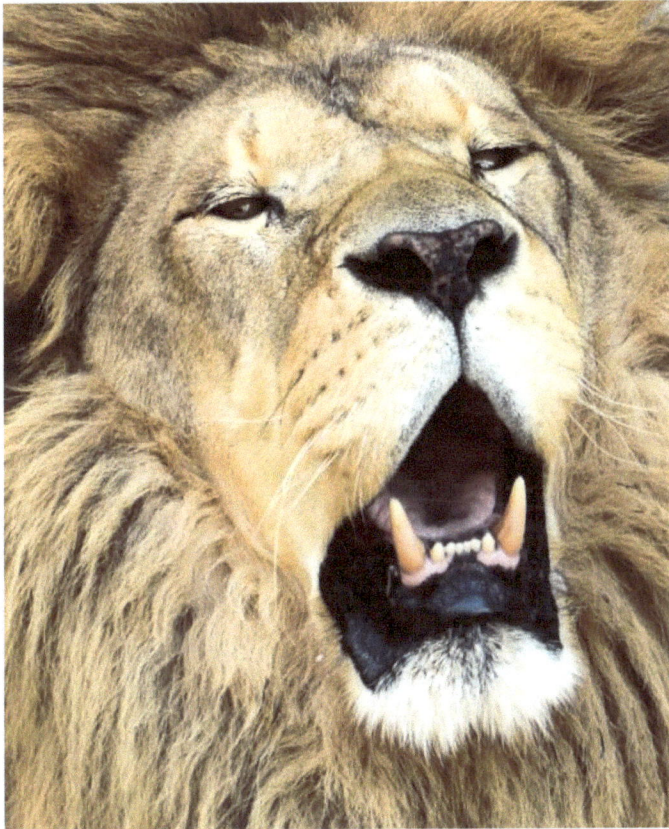

Constipation

"Courage is what it takes to stand up and speak; courage is also what it takes to sit down and listen."

~Sir Winston Churchill

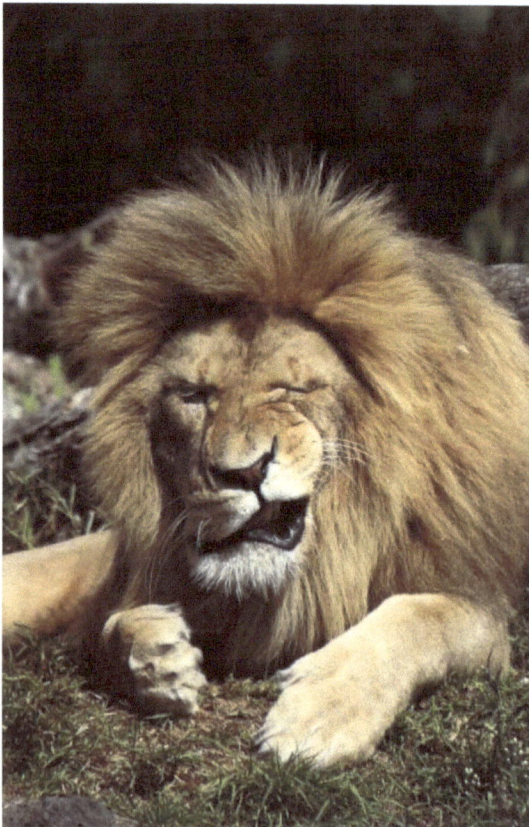

Loss of intimacy

"The best thing to hold onto in life is each other."

~Audrey Hepburn

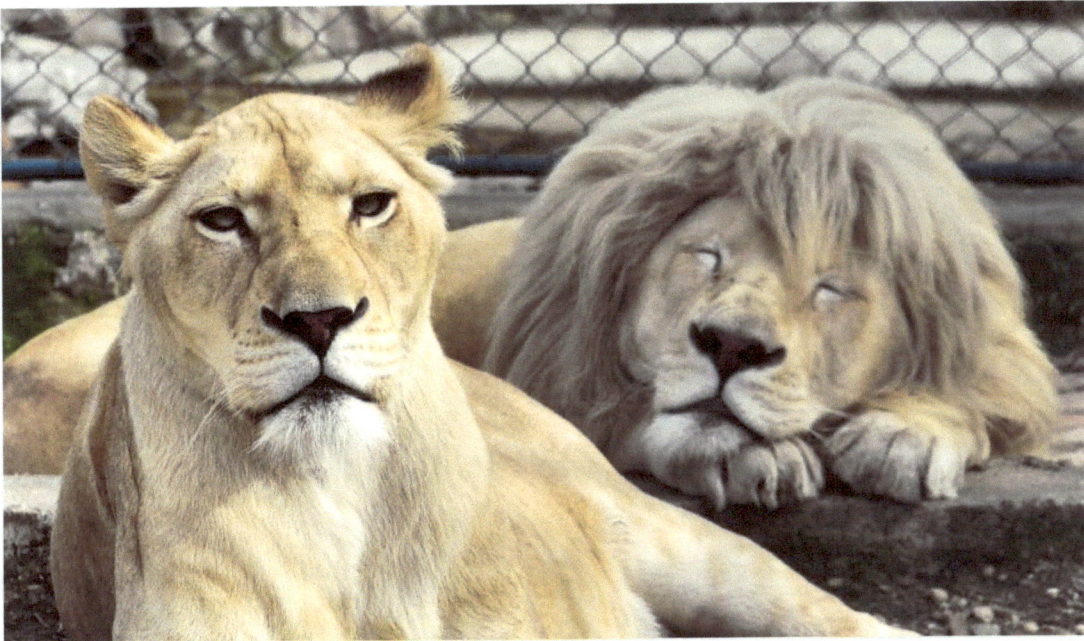

Depression

"To him that waits all things reveal themselves,
provided that he has the courage not to deny,
in the darkness, what he has seen in the light."

~Coventry Patmore

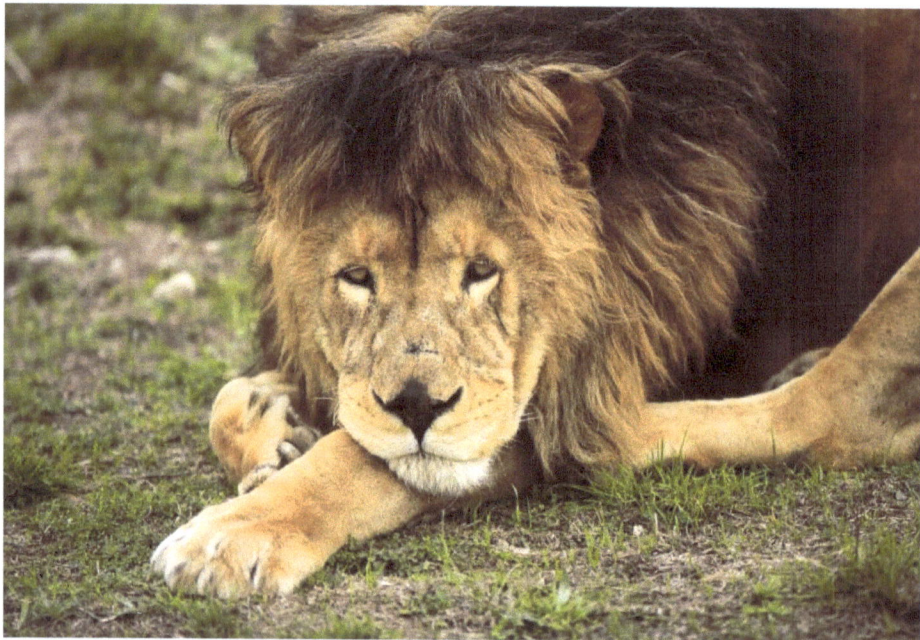

Total exhaustion

"Courage doesn't always roar. Sometimes courage is the little voice at the end of the day that says 'I'll try again tomorrow'."

~Mary Anne Radmacher

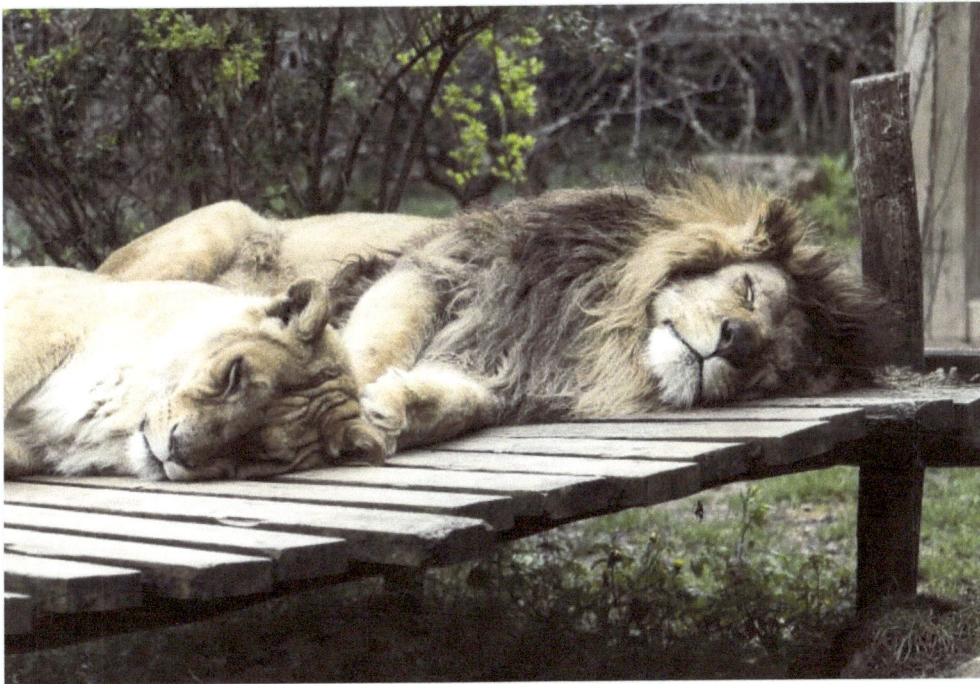

Shaking

"True courage is being afraid and going ahead and doing your job anyhow, that's what courage is."

~Norman Schwarzkopf

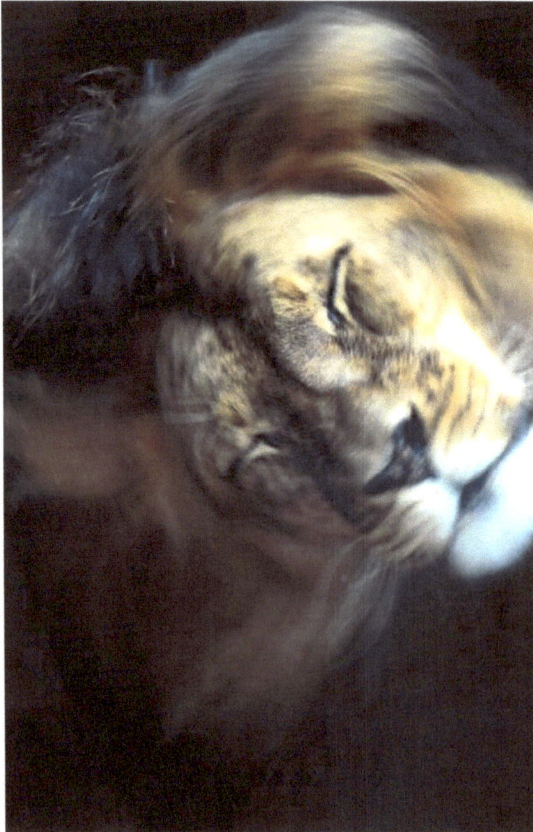

Dry skin and Itchiness

"Courage conquers all things; it even gives strength to the body."

~Ovid

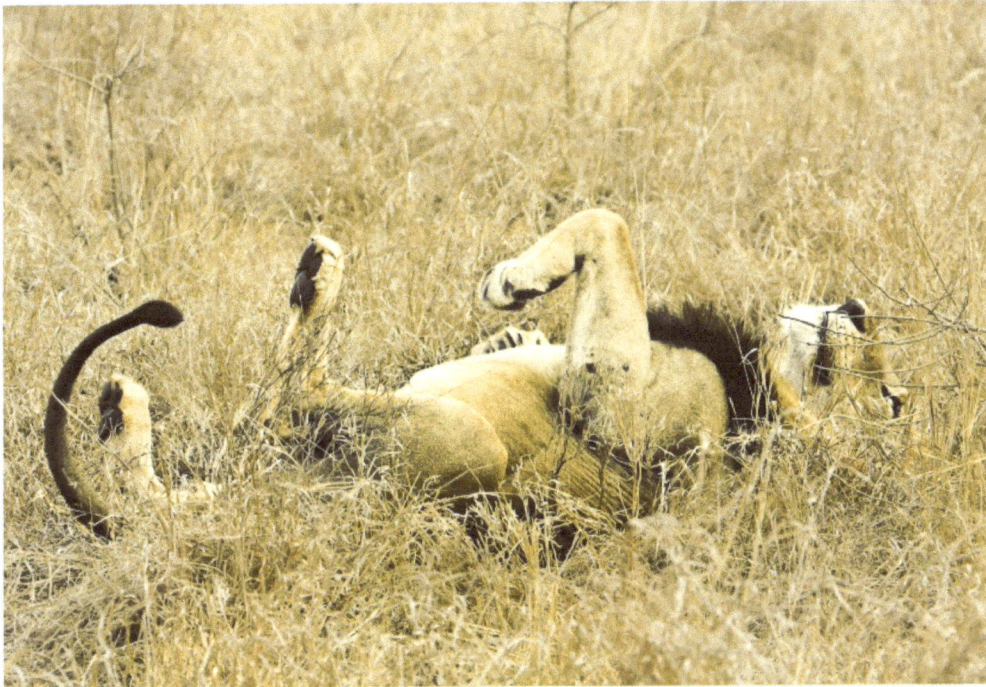

Excessive energy

"In terms of fitness and battling through cancer, exercise helps you stay strong physically and mentally."

~Grete Waitz

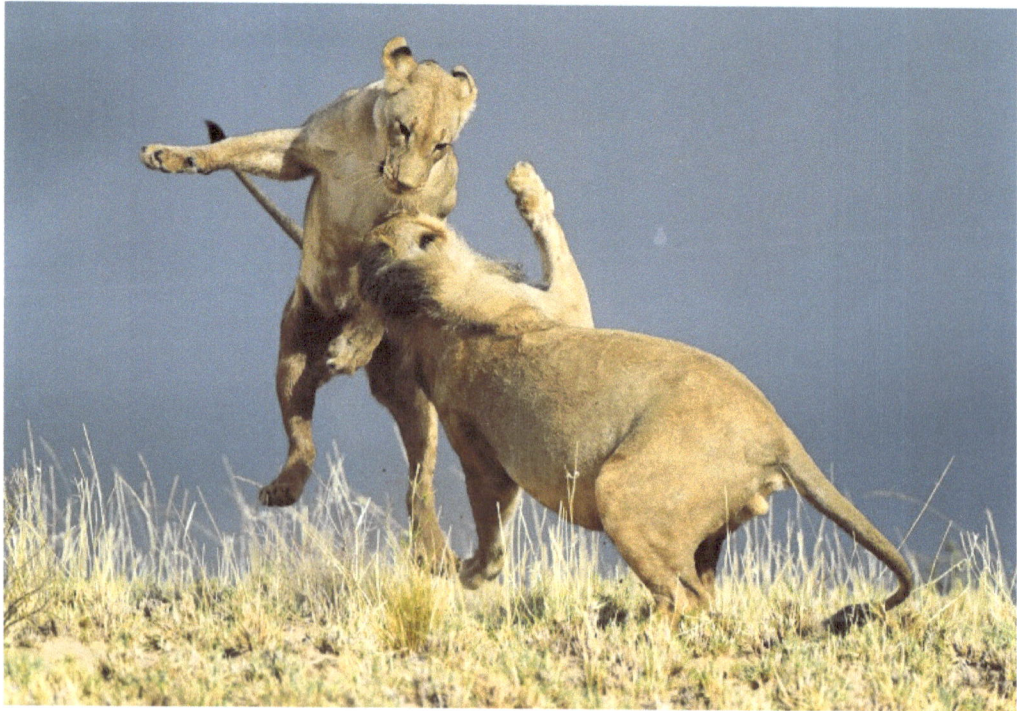

Incessant talking

"Speaking with kindness creates confidence,
thinking with kindness creates profoundness,
giving with kindness creates love."

~Lao Tzu

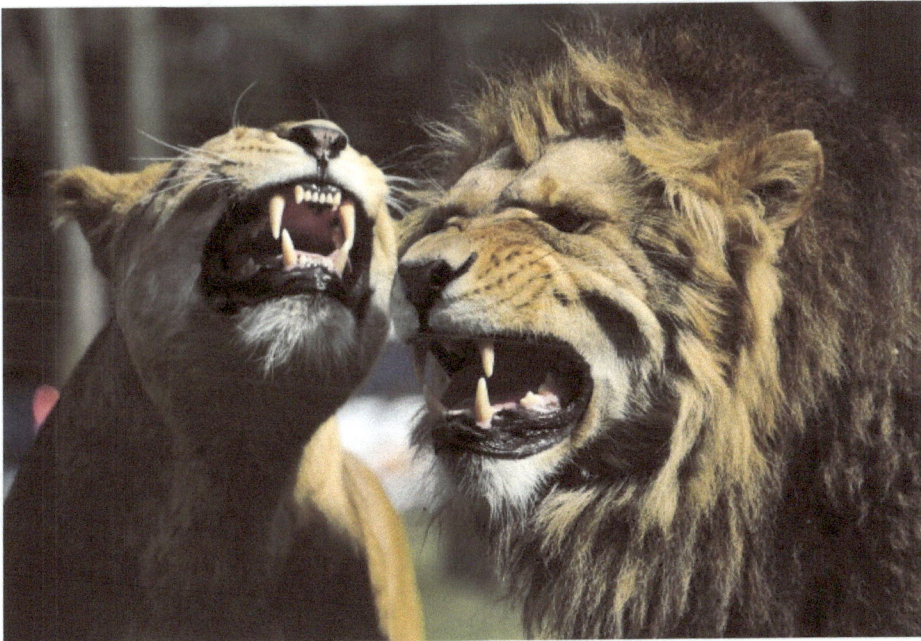

Crashing

"Courage is found in unlikely places."

~J. R. R. Tolkien

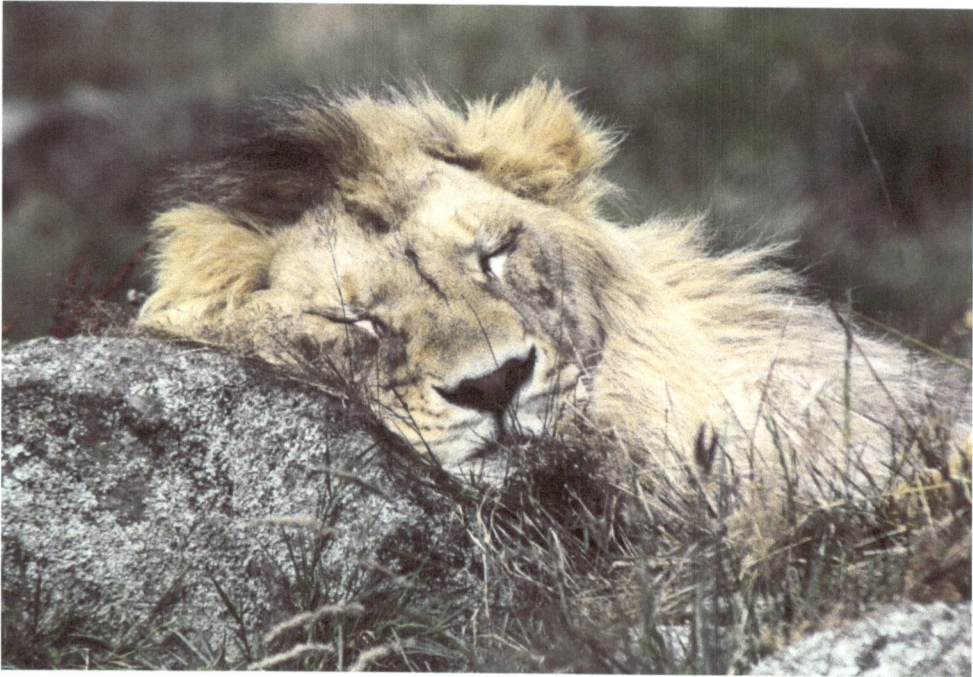

Increased appetite

"Let food be thy medicine and medicine be thy food."

~Hippocrates

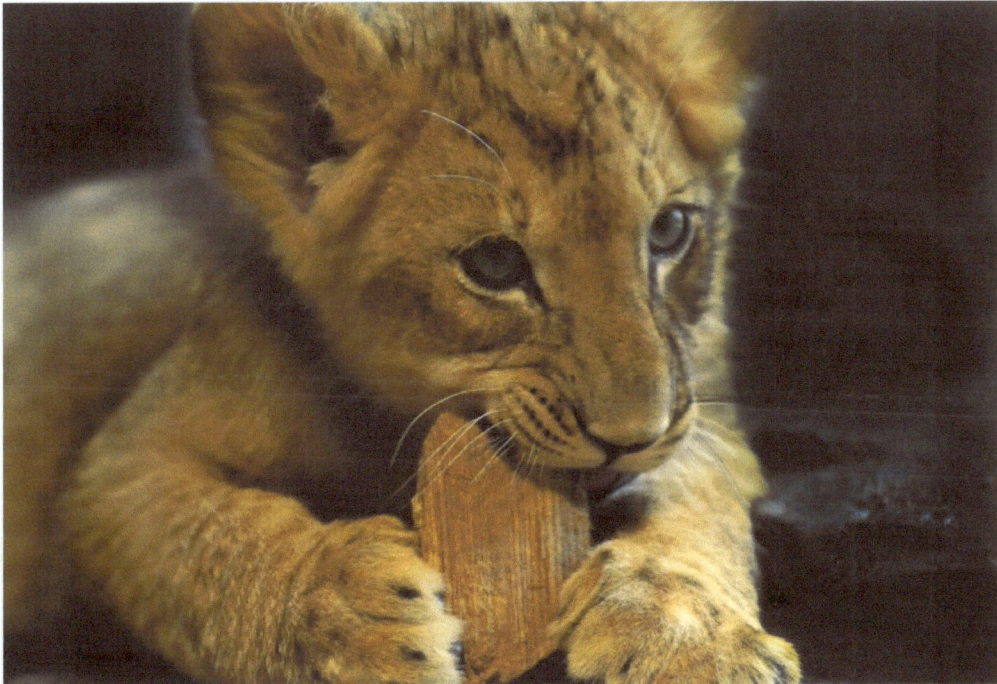

Swelling and Puffiness

"All human wisdom is summed up in two words: wait and hope."

~Alexandre Dumas

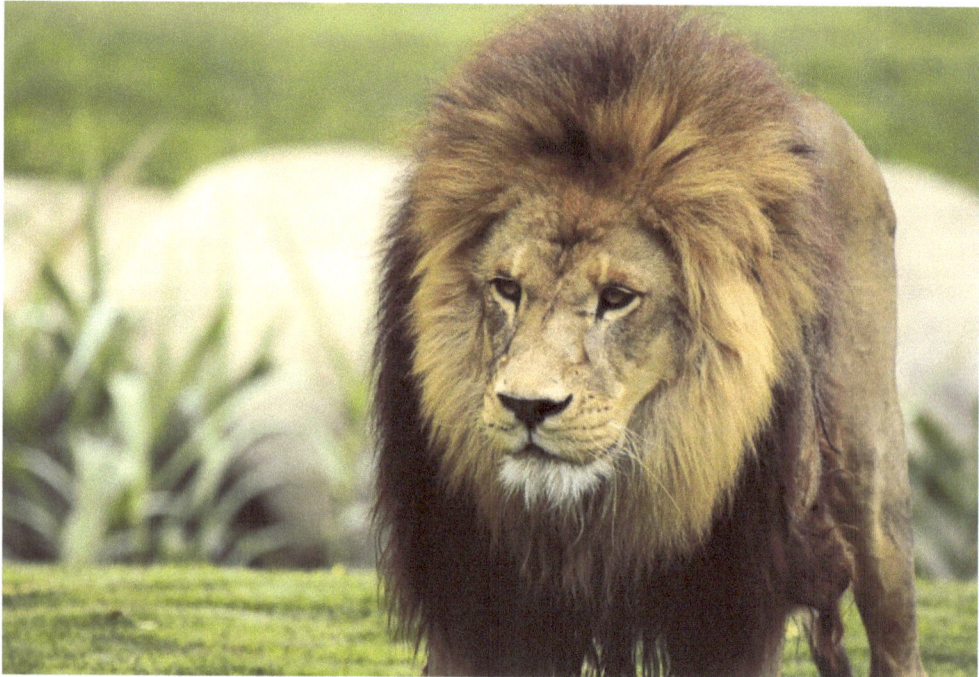

Prolonged memory loss
(mental cloudiness)

"Courage is knowing what not to fear."

~Plato

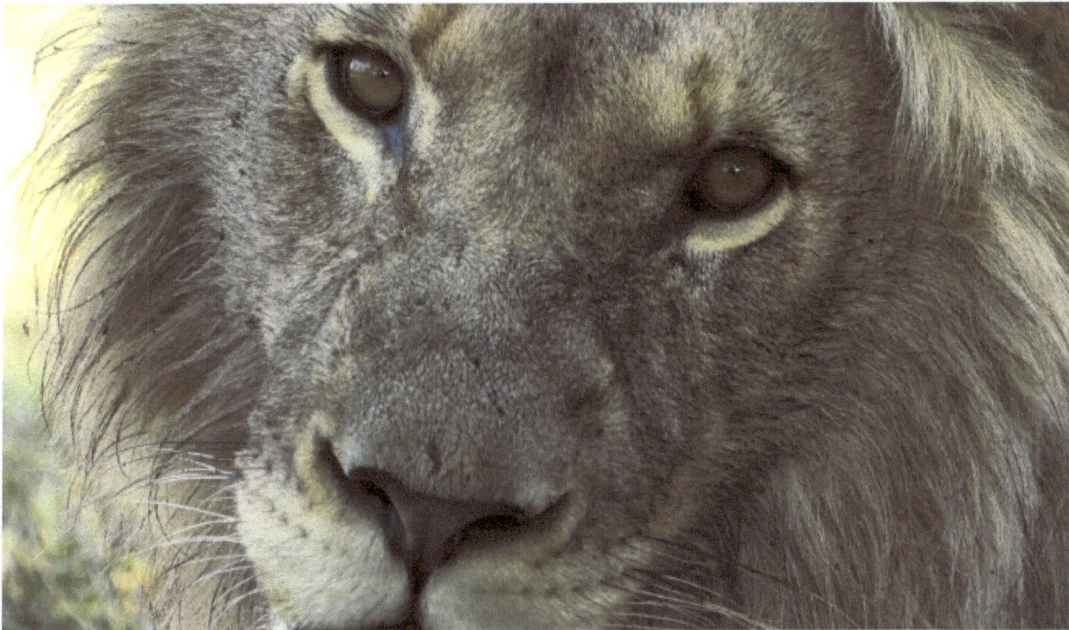

Prolonged neuropathy

"Find a place inside where there's joy, and the joy will burn out the pain."

~Joseph Campbell

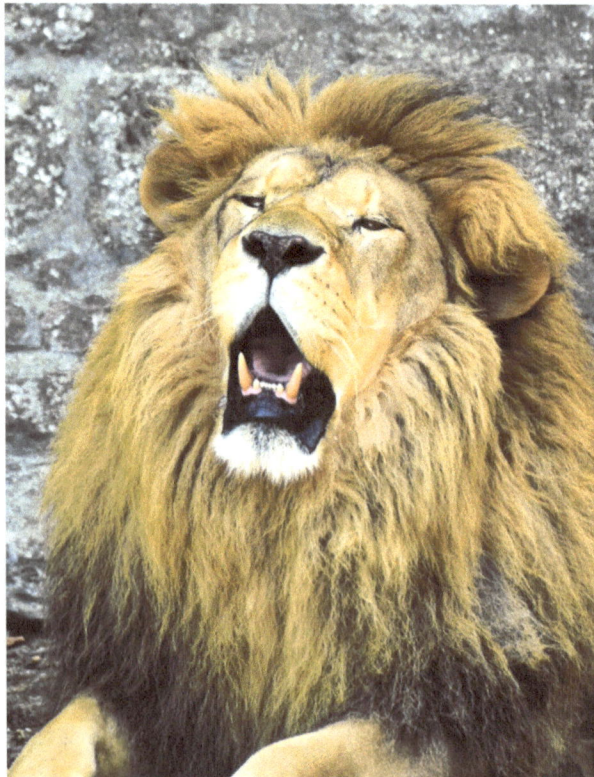

Waiting for treatment to be done

"The only courage that matters is the kind that gets you from one moment to the next."

~Mignon McLaughlin

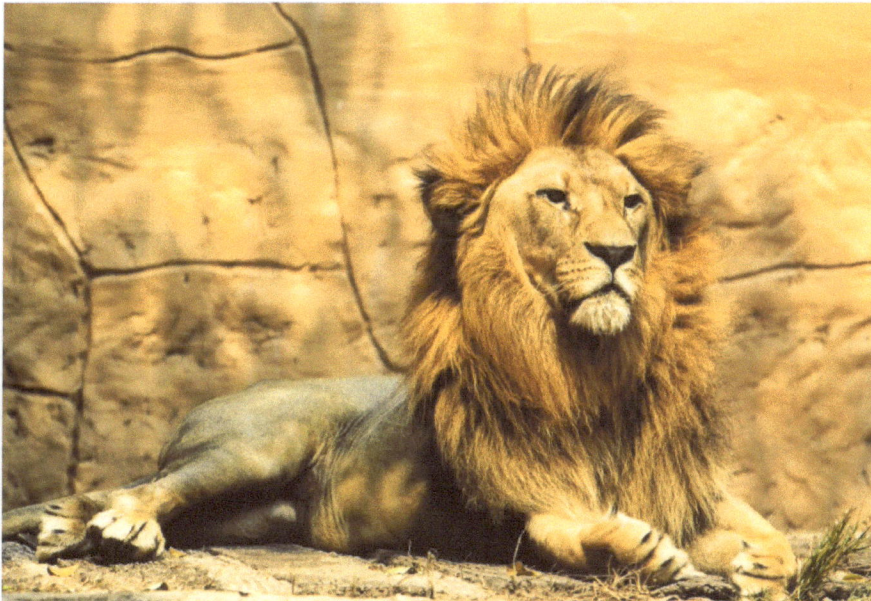

You're entitled..........

……. to your feelings

Feeling sorry for yourself

"Keep courage. Whatever you do, do not feel sorry for yourself. You will win in a great age of opportunity."

~Richard L. Evans

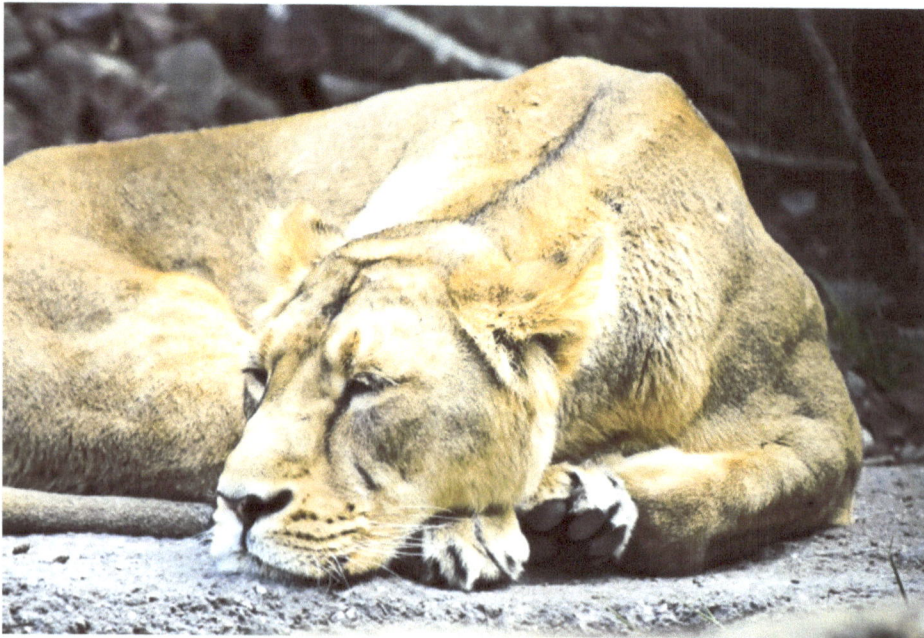

Feeling "unreal" or detached

"Sometimes the biggest act of courage is a small one."

~Lauren Raffo

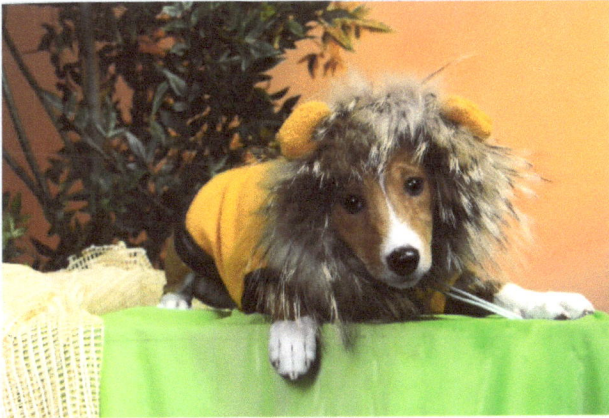
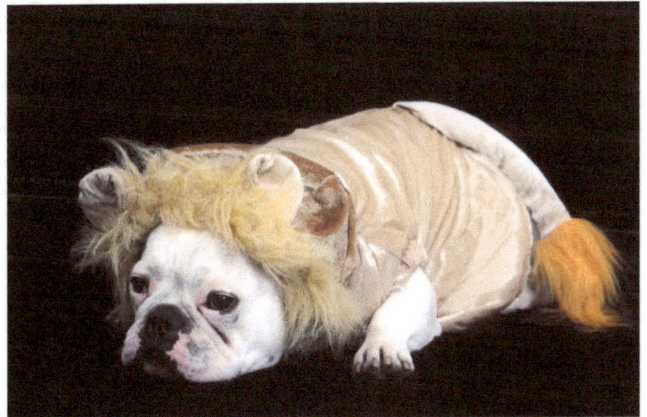

Feeling isolated

"Keep your face always toward the sunshine,
and shadows will fall behind you."

~Walt Whitman

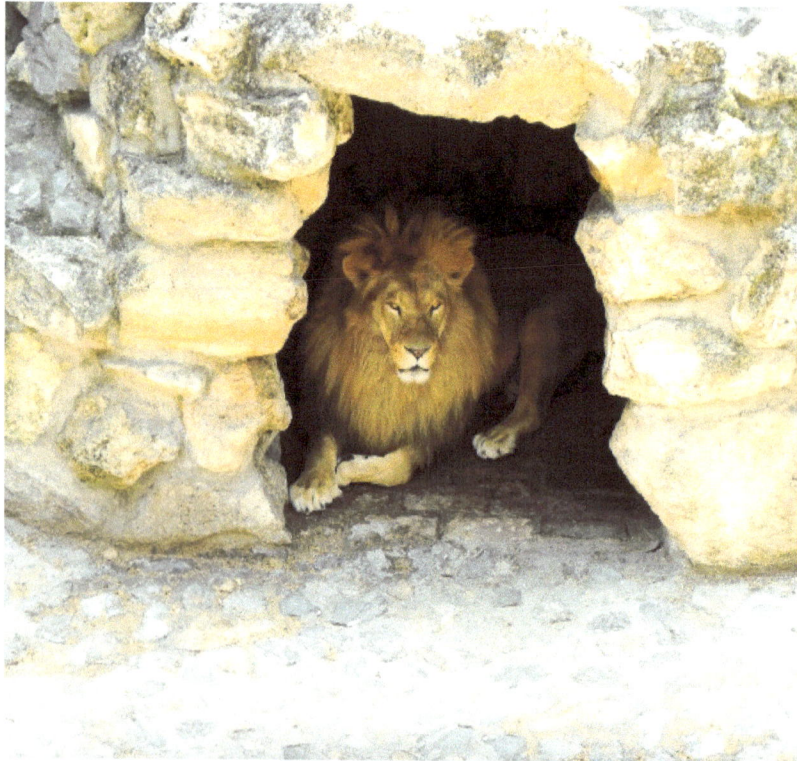

Feeling angry

"Courage is grace under pressure."

~Ernest Hemingway

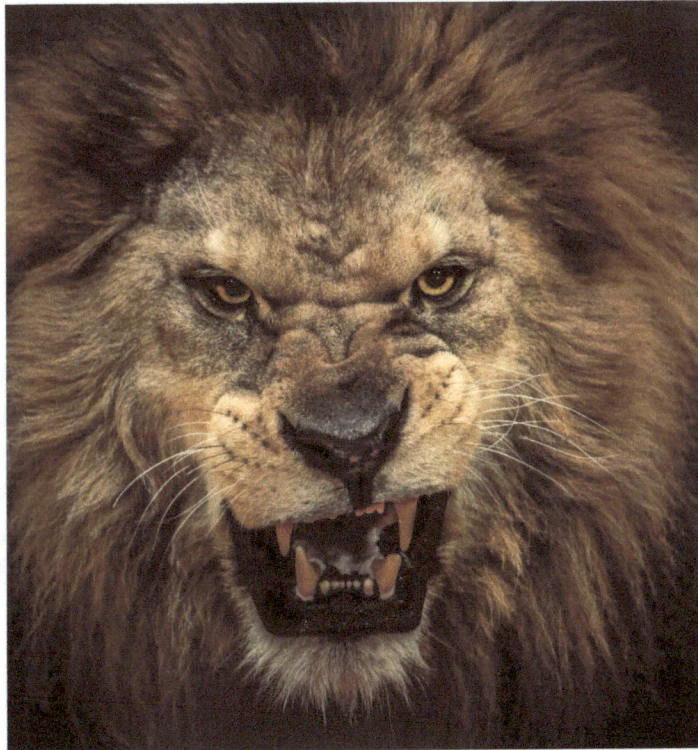

Feeling anxious

"There is no medicine like hope, no incentive so great, and no tonic so powerful as expectation of something tomorrow."

~Orison Swett Marden

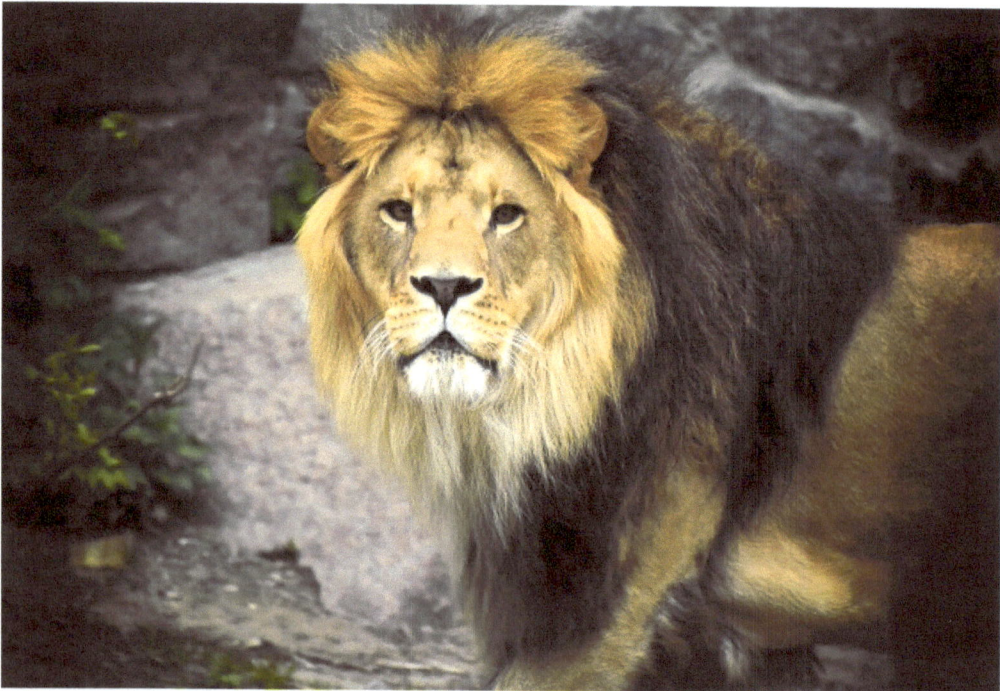

Panic attacks

"Courage is never to let your actions be influenced by your fears."

~Arthur Koestler

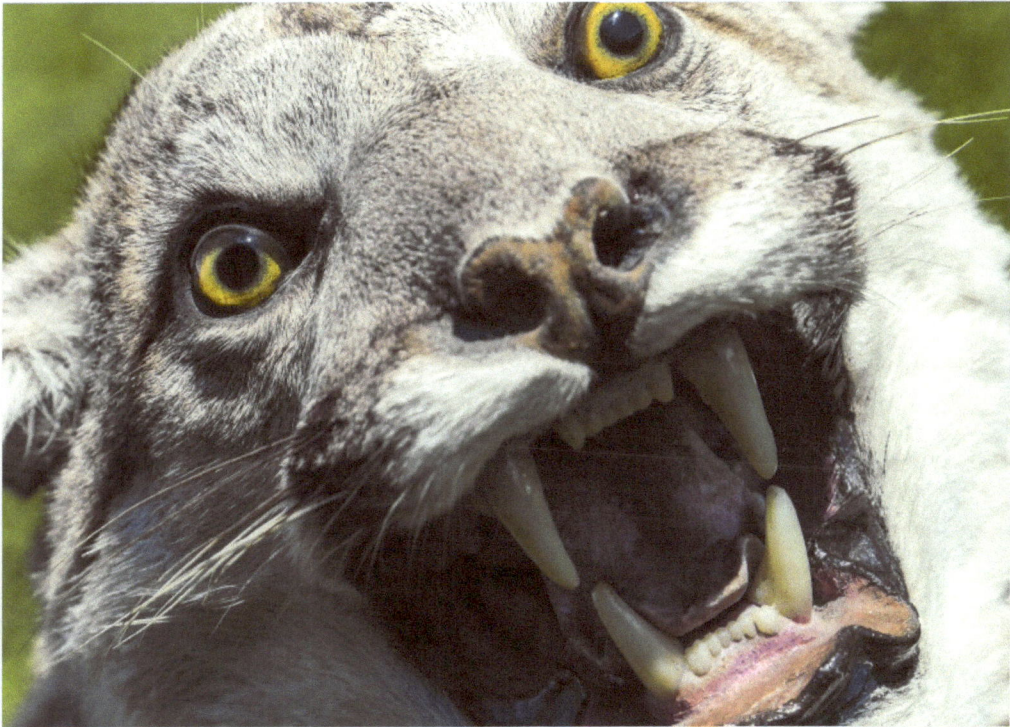

Loss of independence

"Walking with a friend in the dark is better than walking alone in the light."

~Helen Keller

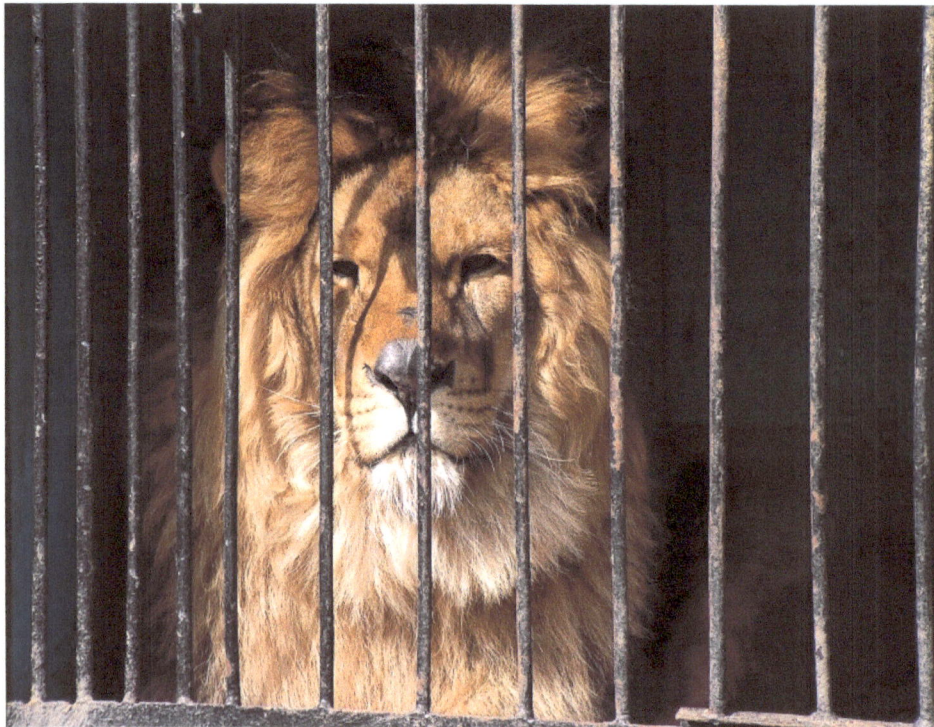

Mood swings
(especially anger)

"There is a thin line that separates laughter and pain, comedy and tragedy, humor and hurt."

~Erma Bombeck

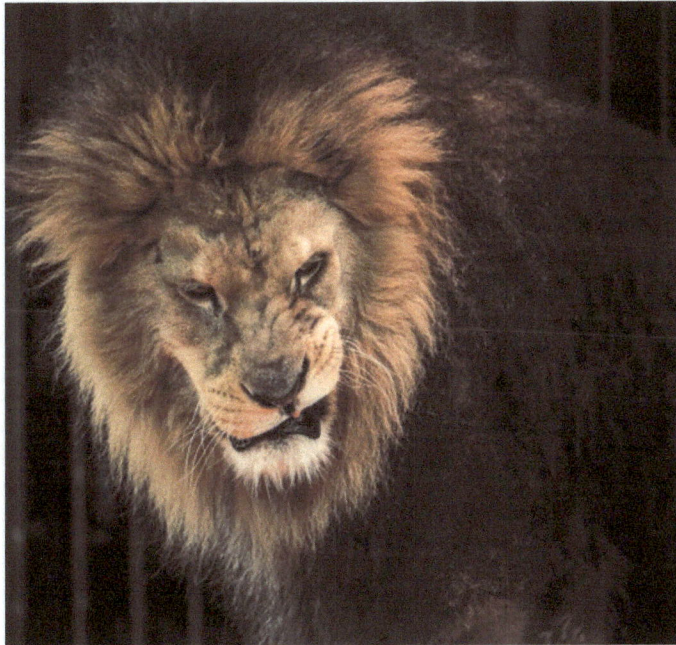

Complain as much as you want......

"We don't develop courage by being happy every day.   We develop it by surviving difficult times and challenging adversity."

~Barbara de Angelis

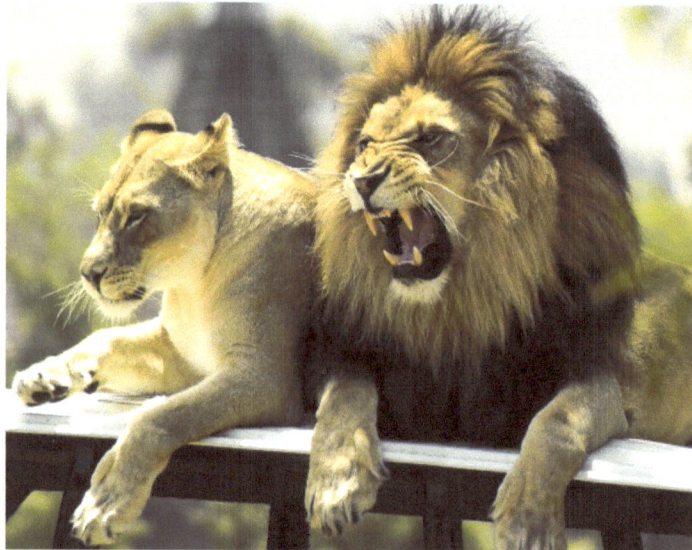

but remember, treatments are only temporary

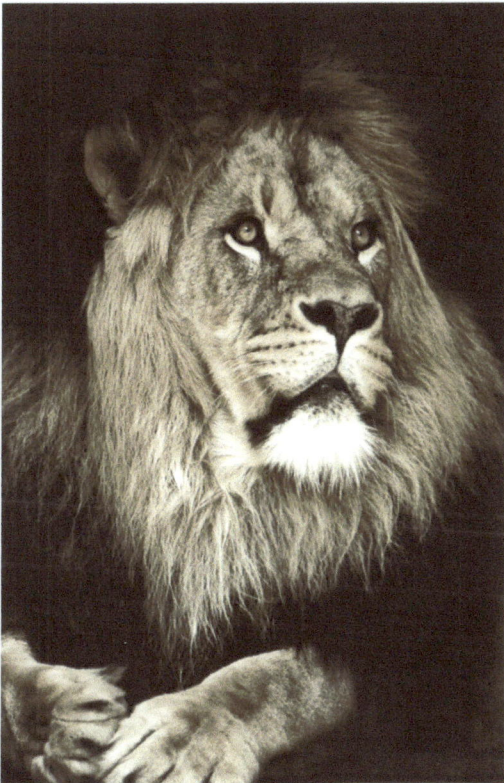

"Let me not pray to be sheltered from dangers, but to be fearless in facing them.

Let me not beg for the stilling of my pain, but for the heart to conquer it."

~Rabindranath Tagore

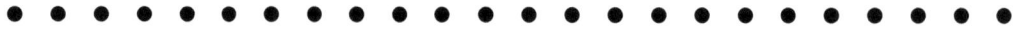

…….on the bright side

There are wonderful doctors

"The good physician treats the disease; the great physician treats the patient who has the disease."

~Sir William Osler

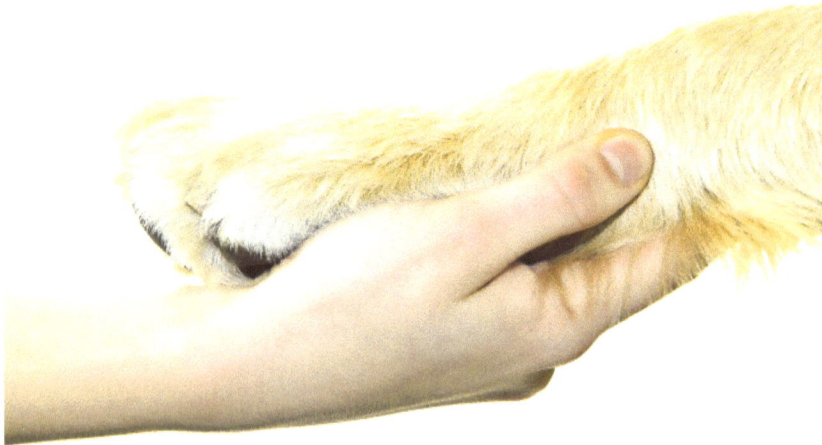

and compassionate caregivers

"The purpose of human life is to serve, and to show compassion and the will to help others."

~Albert Schweitzer

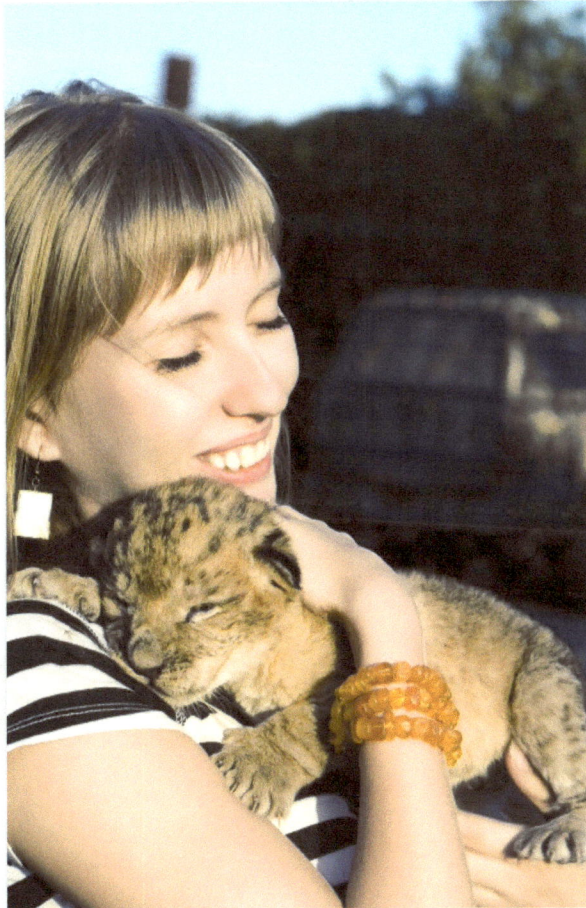

Fellow patients and support groups will help you

"As we express our gratitude, we must never forget that the highest appreciation is not to utter words, but to live by them."

~John F. Kennedy

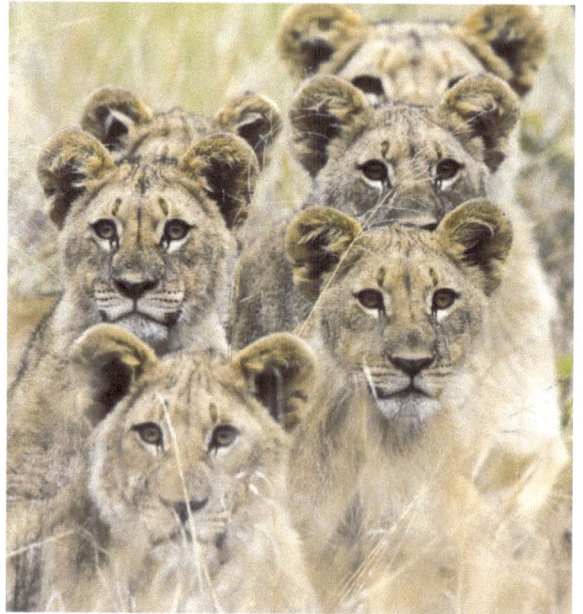

There is love and laughter

"I think laughter may be a form of courage. As humans we sometimes stand tall and look into the sun and laugh, and I think we are never more brave than when we do that."

~Linda Ellerbee

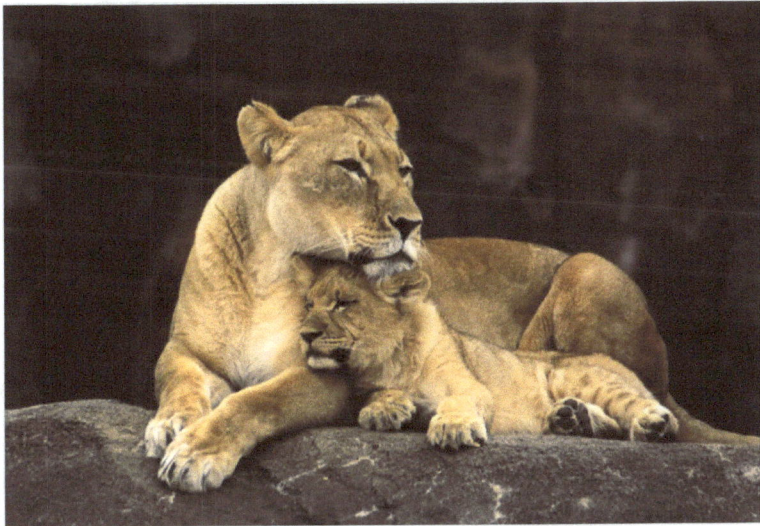

Pamper yourself

"Courage ought to have eyes as well as arms."

~Henry George Bohn

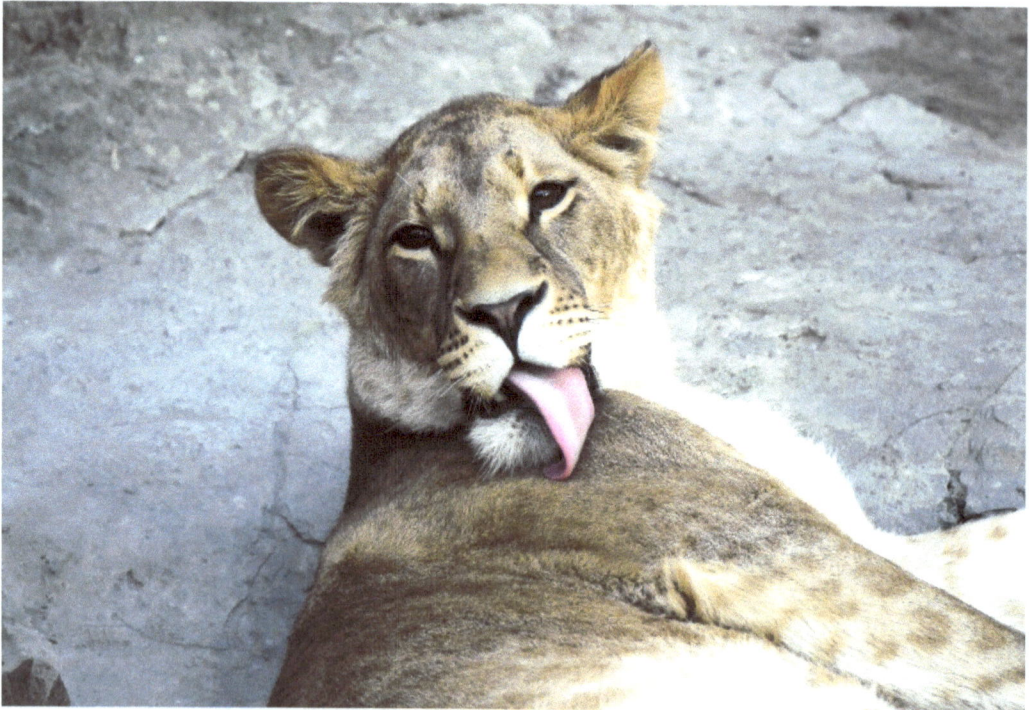

Plenty of scarves
and hats

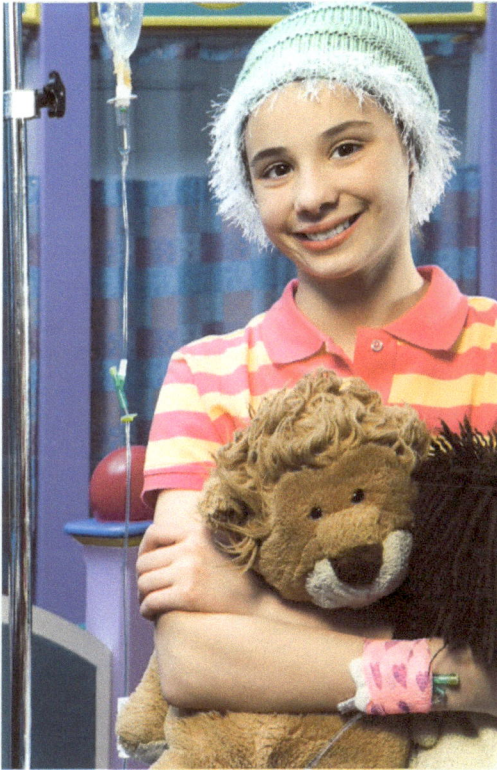

"Optimism is essential to achievement and it is also the foundation of courage and true progress."

~Nicholas M. Butler

Keep your chin up and pray

"God grant me the courage not to give up what I think is right even though I think it is hopeless."

~Chester W. Nimitz

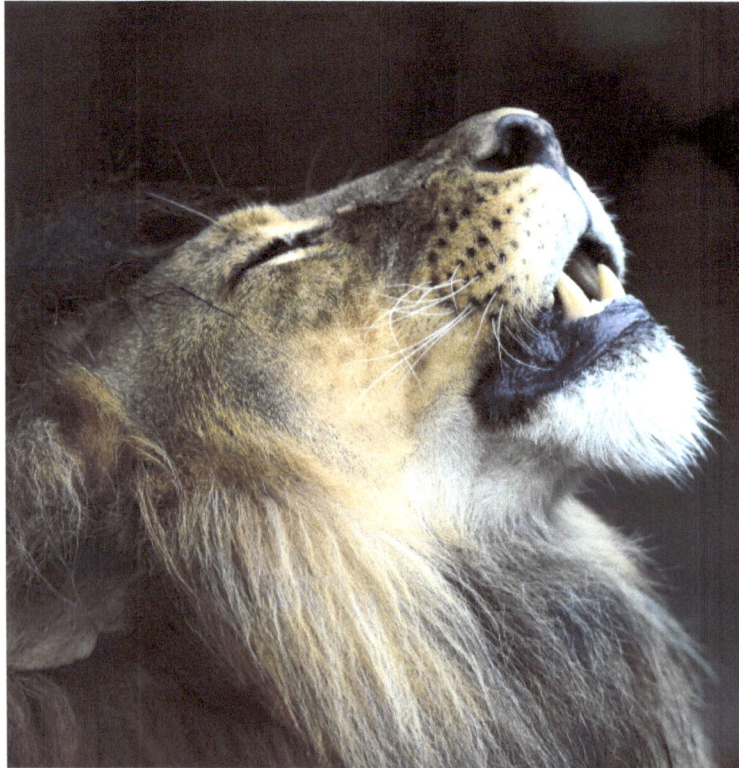

You're stronger than you realize

"Courage crawls atop fear and screams loud its mighty victory."

~Terri Guillemets

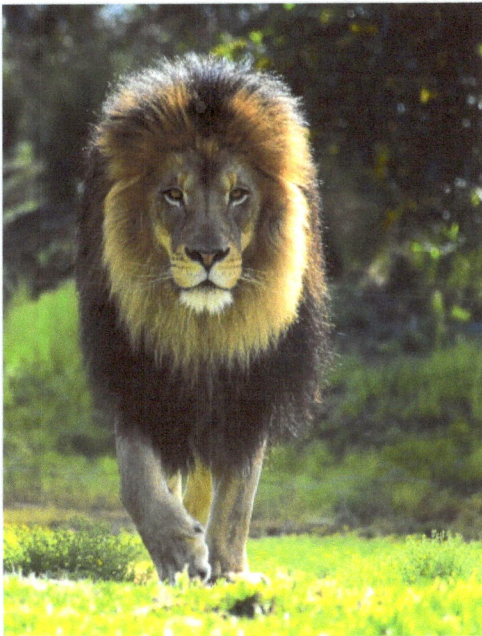

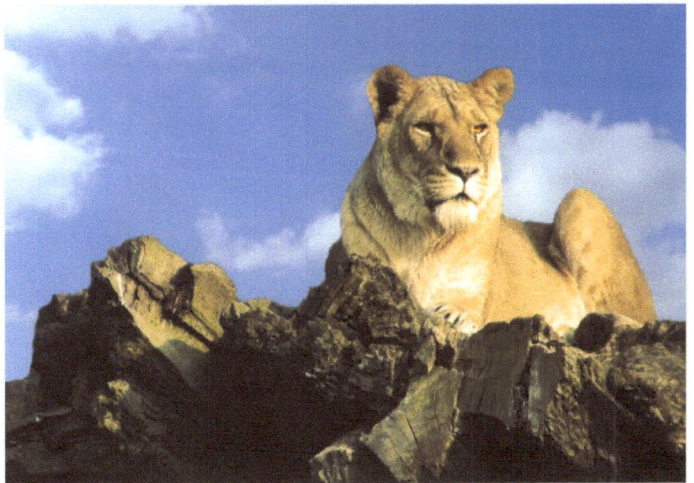

Give back to help others

"No one has yet computed how many imaginary triumphs are silently celebrated by people each year to keep up their courage."

~Henry S. Haskins

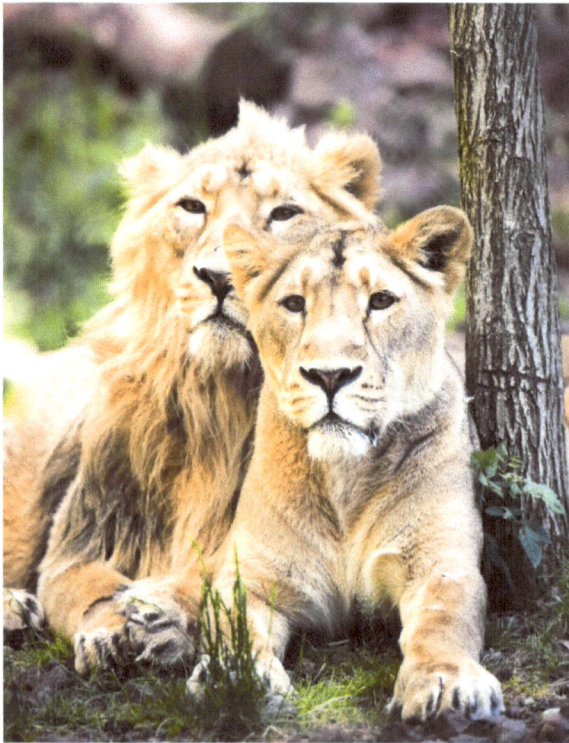

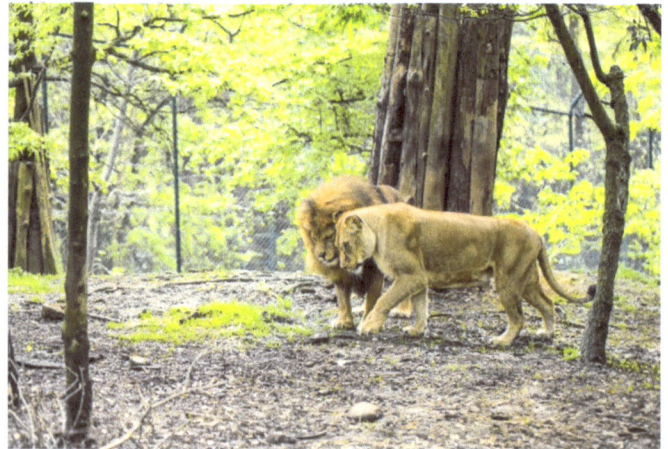

Your courage can inspire others

"A hero is someone who has given his or her life to something bigger than oneself.

~Joseph Campbell

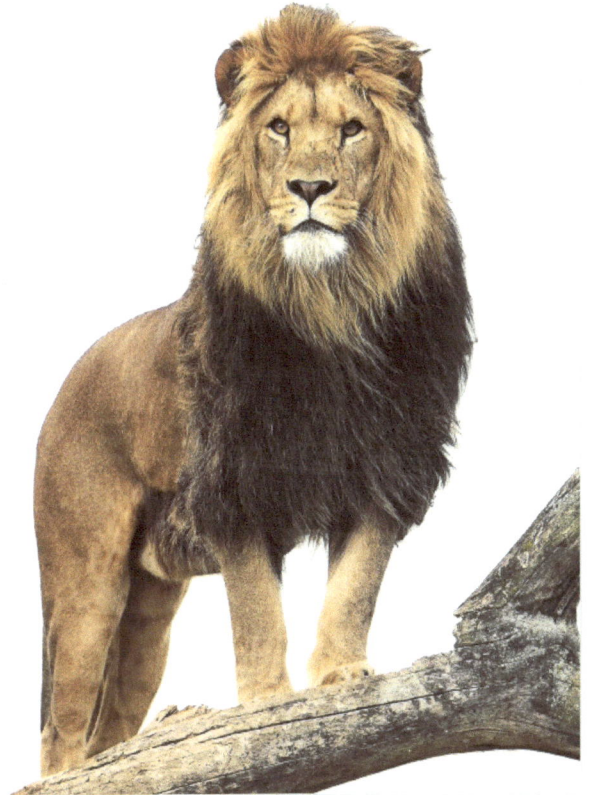

The road to recovery is long

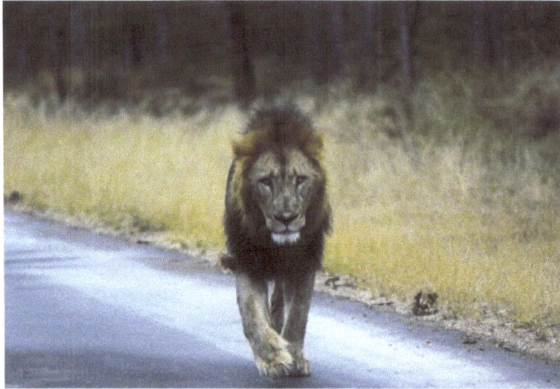

"All you need is a plan, the road map, and the courage to press on to your destination."

~Earl Nightingale

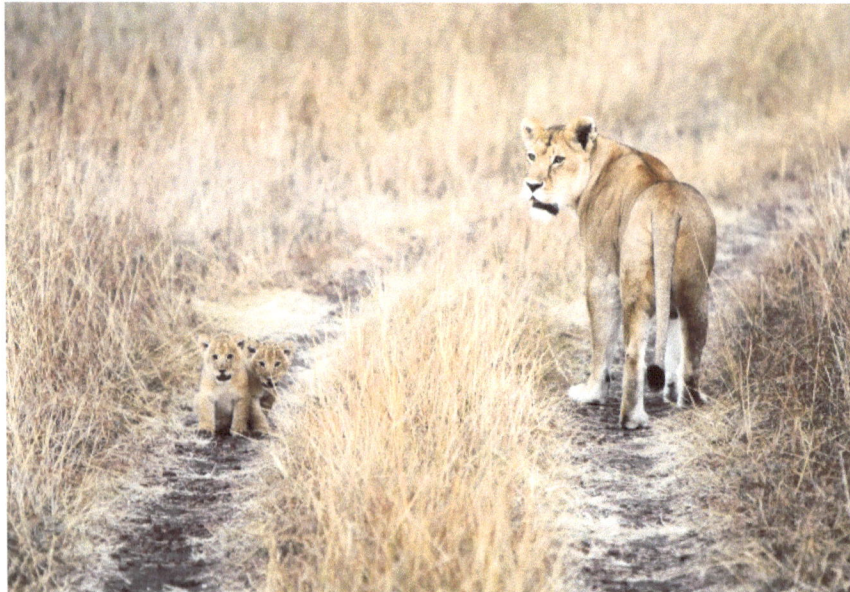

but you're a Survivor

"What I would say to anybody facing any life challenge or disease is that that is courage – to choose life, to keep looking at what's good."

~Debbie Ford

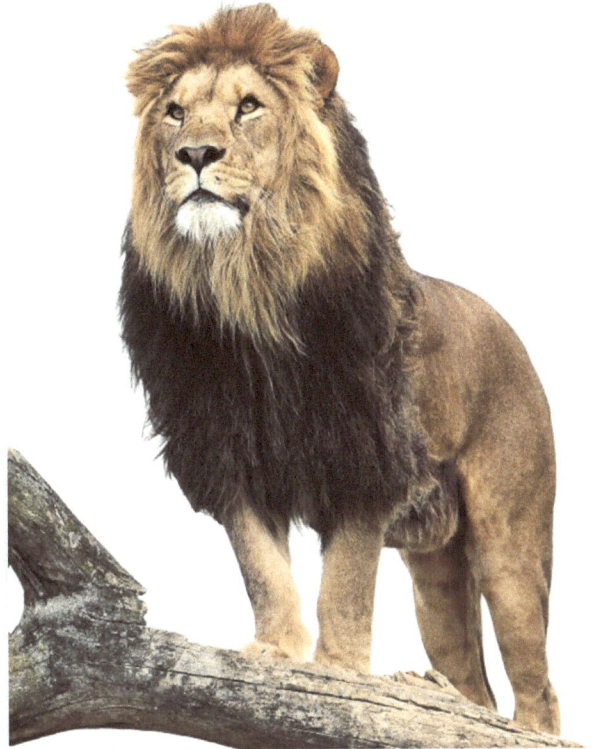

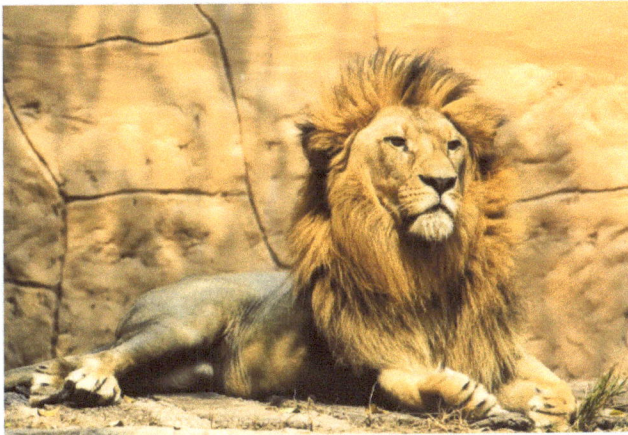

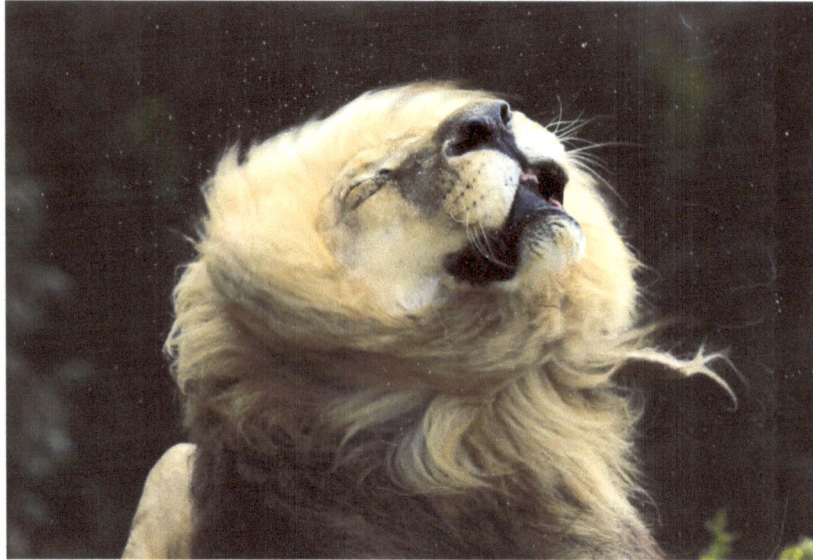

"True courage is like a kite; a contrary wind raises it higher."

~John Petit-Senn

Courage takes on many forms and is a necessary virtue for living a satisfying life. It is an attribute of good character that makes one worthy of respect.

Everyone has a certain level of courage which allows them to face their fears and life challenges; without it, we lose the ability to face risk and may never be able to achieve anything.

Even though life will deliver many moments of despair, they can be overcome with courage, hope, a little patience, and a positive attitude.

It is that positive attitude and courage that will lead the way towards healing and recovery.

Words of encouragement

Words of encouragement

Proceeds from the sale of this book benefit patient programs and cancer research.

Thank you for your support.